MILNE

Springer Series in Statistics

Advisors:
P. Bickel, P. Diggle, S. Fienberg, K. Krickeberg,
I. Olkin, N. Wermuth, S. Zeger

Springer
London
Berlin
Heidelberg
New York
Hong Kong
Milan
Paris
Tokyo

Springer Series in Statistics

Andersen/Borgan/Gill/Keiding: Statistical Models Based on Counting Processes.
Atkinson/Riani: Robust Diagnostic Regression Analysis.
Berger: Statistical Decision Theory and Bayesian Analysis, 2nd edition.
Borg/Groenen: Modern Multidimensional Scaling: Theory and Applications
Brockwell/Davis: Time Series: Theory and Methods, 2nd edition.
Chan/Tong: Chaos: A Statistical Perspective.
Chen/Shao/Ibrahim: Monte Carlo Methods in Bayesian Computation.
David/Edwards: Annotated Readings in the History of Statistics.
Devroye/Lugosi: Combinatorial Methods in Density Estimation.
Efromovich: Nonparametric Curve Estimation: Methods, Theory, and Applications.
Eggermont/LaRiccia: Maximum Penalized Likelihood Estimation, Volume I: Density Estimation.
Fahrmeir/Tutz: Multivariate Statistical Modelling Based on Generalized Linear Models, 2nd edition.
Fan/Yao: Nonlinear Time Series: Nonparametric and Parametric Methods.
Farebrother: Fitting Linear Relationships: A History of the Calculus of Observations 1750-1900.
Federer: Statistical Design and Analysis for Intercropping Experiments, Volume I: Two Crops.
Federer: Statistical Design and Analysis for Intercropping Experiments, Volume II: Three or More Crops.
Ghosh/Ramamoorthi: Bayesian Nonparametrics.
Glaz/Naus/Wallenstein: Scan Statistics.
Good: Permutation Tests: A Practical Guide to Resampling Methods for Testing Hypotheses, 2nd edition.
Gouriéroux: ARCH Models and Financial Applications.
Gu: Smoothing Spline ANOVA Models.
Györfi/Kohler/Krzyżak/ Walk: A Distribution-Free Theory of Nonparametric Regression.
Haberman: Advanced Statistics, Volume I: Description of Populations.
Hall: The Bootstrap and Edgeworth Expansion.
Härdle: Smoothing Techniques: With Implementation in S.
Harrell: Regression Modeling Strategies: With Applications to Linear Models, Logistic Regression, and Survival Analysis
Hart: Nonparametric Smoothing and Lack-of-Fit Tests.
Hastie/Tibshirani/Friedman: The Elements of Statistical Learning: Data Mining, Inference, and Prediction
Hedayat/Sloane/Stufken: Orthogonal Arrays: Theory and Applications.
Heyde: Quasi-Likelihood and its Application: A General Approach to Optimal Parameter Estimation.
Huet/Bouvier/Gruet/Jolivet: Statistical Tools for Nonlinear Regression: A Practical Guide with S-PLUS Examples.
Ibrahim/Chen/Sinha: Bayesian Survival Analysis.
Jolliffe: Principal Component Analysis.

(continued after index)

Stuart Coles

An Introduction to Statistical Modeling of Extreme Values

With 77 Illustrations

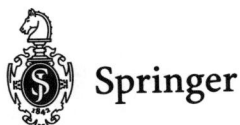 Springer

Stuart Coles
Department of Mathematics
University of Bristol
University Walk
Bristol
BS8 1TW
UK
stuart.coles@bristol.ac.uk

British Library Cataloguing in Publication Data
Coles, Stuart
 An introduction to statistical modeling of extreme values.
 - (Springer series in statistics)
 1. Extreme value theory. 2. Mathematical statistics
 I. Title
 519.5
ISBN 1852334592

Library of Congress Cataloging-in-Publication Data
Coles, Stuart.
 An introduction to statistical modeling of extreme values. / Stuart Coles.
   p. cm. -- (Springer series in statistics)
 Includes bibliographical references and index.
 ISBN 1-85233-459-2 (alk. paper)
 1. Extreme value theory. I. Title. II. Series.
QA273.6.C63 2001
519.2'4—dc21   2001042666

Apart from any fair dealing for the purposes of research or private study, or criticism or review, as permitted under the Copyright, Designs and Patents Act 1988, this publication may only be reproduced, stored or transmitted, in any form or by any means, with the prior permission in writing of the publishers, or in the case of reprographic reproduction in accordance with the terms of licences issued by the Copyright Licensing Agency. Enquiries concerning reproduction outside those terms should be sent to the publishers.

ISBN 1-85233-459-2 Springer-Verlag London Berlin Heidelberg
Springer-Verlag is a part of Springer Science+Business Media
springeronline.com

© Springer-Verlag London Limited 2001
Printed in Great Britain
3rd printing 2004

The use of registered names, trademarks etc. in this publication does not imply, even in the absence of a specific statement, that such names are exempt from the relevant laws and regulations and therefore free for general use.

The publisher makes no representation, express or implied, with regard to the accuracy of the information contained in this book and cannot accept any legal responsibility or liability for any errors or omissions that may be made.

Typesetting: Camera ready by the author
Printed and bound at the Athenæum Press Ltd., Gateshead, Tyne & Wear
12/3830-5432 Printed on acid-free paper SPIN 11012382

To Ben and Jodie

Preface

Extreme value theory is unique as a statistical discipline in that it develops techniques and models for describing the unusual rather than the usual. As an abstract study of random phenomena, the subject can be traced back to the early part of the 20th century. It was not until the 1950's that the methodology was proposed in any serious way for the modeling of genuine physical phenomena. It is no coincidence that early applications of extreme value models were primarily in the field of civil engineering: engineers had always been required to design their structures so that they would withstand the forces that might reasonably be expected to impact upon them. Extreme value theory provided a framework in which an estimate of anticipated forces could be made using historical data.

By definition, extreme values are scarce, meaning that estimates are often required for levels of a process that are much greater than have already been observed. This implies an extrapolation from observed levels to unobserved levels, and extreme value theory provides a class of models to enable such extrapolation. In lieu of an empirical or physical basis, asymptotic argument is used to generate the extreme value models. It is easy to be cynical about this strategy, arguing that extrapolation of models to unseen levels requires a leap of faith, even if the models have an underlying asymptotic rationale. There is no simple defense against this criticism, except to say that applications demand extrapolation, and that it is better to use techniques that have a rationale of some sort. This argument is well understood and, notwithstanding objections to the general principle of extrapolation, there are no serious competitor models to those provided by extreme value theory. But there is less common agreement about the statistical methodology with which to infer such models. In this book we adopt a likelihood-based approach, arguing that this affords a framework in which models can be adapted to the types of non-homogeneous patterns of extreme value variation observed in genuine datasets. Other advantages include the ease with which all relevant information can be incorporated into an inference and the facility to quantify uncertainties in estimation.

There are many excellent texts on extreme value theory, covering both probabilistic and statistical aspects. Among these, Gumbel's *Statistics of Extremes* was pivotal in promoting extreme value theory as a tool for modeling the extremal behavior of observed physical processes. Of different emphasis, but similar impact, is *Extremes and Related Properties of Random Sequences and Processes* by Leadbetter, Lindgren and Rootzén. Their arguments greatly advanced the applicability of extreme value techniques in two fundamental ways: first, by the relaxation of classical arguments from independent variables to stationary sequences; second, by the development of broader characterizations of extremal behavior than had previously been given. The aim of the present text is to complement the earlier works with a contemporary statistical view of the discipline.

This book is intended for both statisticians and non-statisticians alike. It is hoped, in particular, that it will appeal to practitioners of extreme value modeling with limited statistical expertise. The mathematical level is elementary, and detailed mathematical proof is usually sacrificed in favor of heuristic argument. Rather more attention is paid to statistical detail, and many examples are provided by way of illustration. All the computations were carried out using the S-PLUS statistical software program, and corresponding datasets and functions are available via the internet as explained in the Appendix.

A wide variety of examples of extreme value problems and datasets are described in Chapter 1. These are drawn from different fields – oceanography, wind engineering and finance, amongst others – and are used to illustrate the various modeling procedures in subsequent chapters. Chapter 2 gives a brief introduction to general techniques of statistical modeling. This chapter could be skipped by readers with a reasonable statistical knowledge.

The heart of the book is contained in Chapters 3 to 8. These chapters include the classical block maxima models for extremes, threshold exceedance models, extensions to stationary and non-stationary sequences, a point process modeling framework and multivariate extreme value models. Chapter 9 provides a brief introduction to a number of more advanced topics, including Bayesian inference and spatial extremes.

The book has developed from introductory courses on extremes given at the Universities of Lancaster, Bristol, Padova and Lausanne (EPFL). I wrote the first draft of the book while on sabbatical at the University of Padova, and would like to thank especially Paola Bortot for sharing many happy days with me and for inspiring me to work on the book. Thanks are also due to many other people. First and foremost, Jonathan Tawn, for teaching me extreme value theory and for being patient with me when I was slow to learn. I'd like also to acknowledge Richard Smith, both for his direct encouragement, and also for initiating an approach to extreme value modeling that emphasizes the role of contemporary statistical techniques. It is largely the fruits of this methodology that I have tried to set out in this book. Both Richard and Jonathan have also been generous in allowing me to use their own datasets in this book: the data of Examples 1.1, 1.3 and 1.4 were provided by Jonathan; those of Examples 1.2, 1.7 and 1.5 by Richard. I'm grateful also to Jan Heffernan for developing some of the S-PLUS functions used in Chapter 8. The list of people who have helped me in less tangible ways is too long to include here, but I should mention in particular my former colleagues from Lancaster University – Peter Diggle, Mandy Chetwynd, Joe Whittaker and Julia Kelsall amongst others – my former Ph.D. students – Elwyn Powell, Ed Casson, Roberto Iannaccone and Francesco Pauli – and my long-term friends – Katherine Fielding and Dave Walshaw. Finally, the book was carefully read by Anthony Davison, whose very detailed comments have enabled me (hopefully) to improve beyond recognition the version he was subjected to.

Stuart Coles   Bristol

Contents

1 Introduction — 1
- 1.1 Basic Concepts — 1
- 1.2 Examples — 4
- 1.3 Structure of the Book — 13
- 1.4 Further Reading — 16

2 Basics of Statistical Modeling — 18
- 2.1 Introduction — 18
- 2.2 Basic Statistical Concepts — 19
  - 2.2.1 Random Variables and Their Distributions — 19
  - 2.2.2 Families of Models — 21
- 2.3 Multivariate Distributions — 22
- 2.4 Random Processes — 25
  - 2.4.1 Stationary Processes — 25
  - 2.4.2 Markov Chains — 25
- 2.5 Limit Laws — 26
- 2.6 Parametric Modeling — 27
  - 2.6.1 The Parametric Framework — 27
  - 2.6.2 Principles of Estimation — 28
  - 2.6.3 Maximum Likelihood Estimation — 30
  - 2.6.4 Approximate Normality of the Maximum Likelihood Estimator — 31

xii   Contents

		2.6.5	Approximate Inference Using the Deviance Function	33
		2.6.6	Inference Using the Profile Likelihood Function . . .	34
		2.6.7	Model Diagnostics	36
	2.7	Example		38
	2.8	Further Reading		43

3 Classical Extreme Value Theory and Models 45
- 3.1 Asymptotic Models 45
  - 3.1.1 Model Formulation 45
  - 3.1.2 Extremal Types Theorem 46
  - 3.1.3 The Generalized Extreme Value Distribution 47
  - 3.1.4 Outline Proof of the Extremal Types Theorem . . . 49
  - 3.1.5 Examples 51
- 3.2 Asymptotic Models for Minima 52
- 3.3 Inference for the GEV Distribution 54
  - 3.3.1 General Considerations 54
  - 3.3.2 Maximum Likelihood Estimation 55
  - 3.3.3 Inference for Return Levels 56
  - 3.3.4 Profile Likelihood 57
  - 3.3.5 Model Checking 57
- 3.4 Examples 59
  - 3.4.1 Annual Maximum Sea-levels at Port Pirie 59
  - 3.4.2 Glass Fiber Strength Example 64
- 3.5 Model Generalization: the r Largest Order Statistic Model . 66
  - 3.5.1 Model Formulation 66
  - 3.5.2 Modeling the r Largest Order Statistics 68
  - 3.5.3 Venice Sea-level Data 69
- 3.6 Further Reading 72

4 Threshold Models 74
- 4.1 Introduction 74
- 4.2 Asymptotic Model Characterization 75
  - 4.2.1 The Generalized Pareto Distribution 75
  - 4.2.2 Outline Justification for the Generalized Pareto Model 76
  - 4.2.3 Examples 77
- 4.3 Modeling Threshold Excesses 78
  - 4.3.1 Threshold Selection 78
  - 4.3.2 Parameter Estimation 80
  - 4.3.3 Return Levels 81
  - 4.3.4 Threshold Choice Revisited 83
  - 4.3.5 Model Checking 84
- 4.4 Examples 84
  - 4.4.1 Daily Rainfall Data 84
  - 4.4.2 Dow Jones Index Series 86
- 4.5 Further Reading 90

5 Extremes of Dependent Sequences — 92
- 5.1 Introduction — 92
- 5.2 Maxima of Stationary Sequences — 93
- 5.3 Modeling Stationary Series — 97
  - 5.3.1 Models for Block Maxima — 98
  - 5.3.2 Threshold Models — 98
  - 5.3.3 Wooster Temperature Series — 100
  - 5.3.4 Dow Jones Index Series — 103
- 5.4 Further Reading — 104

6 Extremes of Non-stationary Sequences — 105
- 6.1 Model Structures — 105
- 6.2 Inference — 108
  - 6.2.1 Parameter Estimation — 108
  - 6.2.2 Model Choice — 109
  - 6.2.3 Model Diagnostics — 110
- 6.3 Examples — 111
  - 6.3.1 Annual Maximum Sea-levels — 111
  - 6.3.2 Race Time Data — 114
  - 6.3.3 Venice Sea-level Data — 117
  - 6.3.4 Daily Rainfall Data — 119
  - 6.3.5 Wooster Temperature Data — 119
- 6.4 Further Reading — 122

7 A Point Process Characterization of Extremes — 124
- 7.1 Introduction — 124
- 7.2 Basic Theory of Point Processes — 124
- 7.3 A Poisson Process Limit for Extremes — 128
  - 7.3.1 Convergence Law — 128
  - 7.3.2 Examples — 130
- 7.4 Connections with Other Extreme Value Models — 131
- 7.5 Statistical Modeling — 132
- 7.6 Connections with Threshold Excess Model Likelihood — 134
- 7.7 Wooster Temperature Series — 136
- 7.8 Return Level Estimation — 137
- 7.9 r Largest Order Statistic Model — 141
- 7.10 Further Reading — 141

8 Multivariate Extremes — 142
- 8.1 Introduction — 142
- 8.2 Componentwise Maxima — 143
  - 8.2.1 Asymptotic Characterization — 143
  - 8.2.2 Modeling — 147
  - 8.2.3 Example: Annual Maximum Sea-levels — 148
  - 8.2.4 Structure Variables — 150

	8.3	Alternative Representations 153
		8.3.1 Bivariate Threshold Excess Model 154
		8.3.2 Point Process Model 156
		8.3.3 Examples 158
	8.4	Asymptotic Independence 163
	8.5	Further Reading 167

9 Further Topics 169
   9.1 Bayesian Inference 169
       9.1.1 General Theory 169
       9.1.2 Bayesian Inference of Extremes 172
       9.1.3 Example: Port Pirie Annual Maximum Sea-levels . . 173
   9.2 Extremes of Markov Chains 177
   9.3 Spatial Extremes 179
       9.3.1 Max-stable Processes 179
       9.3.2 Latent Spatial Process Models 181
   9.4 Further Reading 182

A Computational Aspects 185

References 195

Index 205

1
Introduction

1.1 Basic Concepts

Extreme value theory has emerged as one of the most important statistical disciplines for the applied sciences over the last 50 years. Extreme value techniques are also becoming widely used in many other disciplines. For example: for portfolio adjustment in the insurance industry; for risk assessment on financial markets; and for traffic prediction in telecommunications. At the time of writing, in the past twelve months alone, applications of extreme value modeling have been published in the fields of alloy strength prediction (Tryon & Cruse, 2000); ocean wave modeling (Dawson, 2000); memory cell failure (McNulty et al., 2000); wind engineering (Harris, 2001); management strategy (Dahan & Mendelson, 2001); biomedical data processing (Roberts, 2000); thermodynamics of earthquakes (Lavenda & Cipollone, 2000); assessment of meteorological change (Thompson et al., 2001); non-linear beam vibrations (Dunne & Ghanbari, 2001); and food science (Kawas & Moreira, 2001).

The distinguishing feature of an extreme value analysis is the objective to quantify the stochastic behavior of a process at unusually large – or small – levels. In particular, extreme value analyses usually require estimation of the probability of events that are more extreme than any that have already been observed. By way of example, suppose that, as part of its design criteria for coastal defense, a sea-wall is required to protect against all sea-levels that it is likely to experience within its projected life span of, say, 100 years. Local data on sea-levels might be available, but for a much shorter period, of say 10 years. The challenge is to estimate what sea-levels might occur over the next 100 years given the 10-year history. Extreme value theory provides a framework that enables extrapolations of this type.

In the absence of empirical or physical guidelines with which to formulate an extrapolation rule, standard models are derived from asymptotic argument. In the simplest case this works as follows. Suppose we denote by $X_1, X_2, \ldots$ the sequence of hourly sea-levels. Then

$$M_n = \max\{X_1, \ldots, X_n\} \tag{1.1}$$

is the maximum sea-level over an "n-observation" period. If the exact statistical behavior of the X_i were known, the corresponding behavior of M_n could be calculated exactly. In practice the behavior of the X_i is unknown, making exact calculations on M_n impossible. However, under suitable assumptions, the approximate behavior of M_n for large values of n follows from detailed limit arguments by letting $n \to \infty$, leading to a family of models that can be calibrated by the observed values of M_n. This approach might be termed the **extreme value paradigm**, since it comprises a principle for model extrapolation based on the implementation of mathematical limits as finite-level approximations. It is easy to object to this procedure on the grounds that, even with the support of asymptotic argument, there is an implicit assumption that the underlying stochastic mechanism of the process being modeled is sufficiently smooth to enable extrapolation to unobserved levels. However, no more credible alternative has been proposed to date.

From the outset it is important to be aware of the limitations implied by adoption of the extreme value paradigm. First, the models are developed using asymptotic arguments, and care is needed in treating them as exact results for finite samples. Second, the models themselves are derived under idealized circumstances, which may not be exact (or even reasonable) for a process under study. Third, the models may lead to a wastage of information when implemented in practice. To make this last point clear, a common way of recording extreme data is to store only the maximum observed value over a specified period, perhaps the annual maximum. This corresponds to (1.1) in which n is the number of observations in a year. Assuming this value of n is large enough, the asymptotic arguments lead to a model that describes the variations in annual maxima from one year to another, and which can be fitted to the observed annual maxima. But in any particular year, additional extreme events may have occurred that are possibly more extreme than the maximum in other years. Because such data are not the annual maximum in the year they arose, they are excluded from the analysis.

All of these points emphasize the importance of statistical implementation as a complement to the development of appropriate models for extremes. Four issues, in particular, need to be considered.

1. **Method of estimation**
   This is the means by which the unknown parameters of a model are inferred on the basis of historical data. Though many different approaches have been proposed for the estimation of extreme value models, we take a singular view and restrict attention to techniques based on the likelihood function. All estimation techniques have their pros and cons, but likelihood-based techniques are unique in their adaptability to model-change. That is, although the estimating equations change if a model is modified, the underlying methodology is essentially unchanged. Mostly, we adopt maximum likelihood, which has a convenient set of "off-the-shelf" large-sample inference properties. In Chapter 9 we also discuss briefly the use of Bayesian inferential techniques.

2. **Quantification of uncertainty**
   In any statistical analysis, estimates are "best guesses" at the truth given the available historical information. It is implicit that other data, equally representative of the true process being studied, would have led to different estimates. Consequently, it is important to complement the estimate of a model with measures of uncertainty due to sampling variability. This is especially so in extreme value modeling, where quite small model changes can be greatly magnified on extrapolation. Despite this, the measurement of uncertainty has often been ignored in extreme value applications. There is some irony in this, as an analysis of extreme values is likely to have more sources of uncertainty than most other statistical analyses. Furthermore, estimation of the uncertainty of extreme levels of a process can be as important a design parameter as an estimate of the level itself. We will see that, by basing inference on the likelihood function, estimates of uncertainty are easily obtained.

3. **Model diagnostics**
   The only justification for extrapolating an extreme value model is the asymptotic basis on which it is derived. However, if a model is found to perform badly in terms of its representation for the extreme values that have already been observed, there is little hope of it working well in extrapolation. For each extreme value model introduced in subsequent chapters, we describe several methods for assessing the goodness-of-fit.

4. **Maximal use of information**
   Though uncertainty is inherent in any statistical model, such uncertainties can be reduced by judicious choices of model and inference, and by the utilization of all sources of information. In an extreme value context, possibilities include the use of alternative models that exploit more data than just block maxima; the use of covariate in-

formation; the construction of multivariate models; and the incorporation of additional sources of knowledge or information into an analysis. Each of these approaches is discussed in subsequent chapters.

1.2 Examples

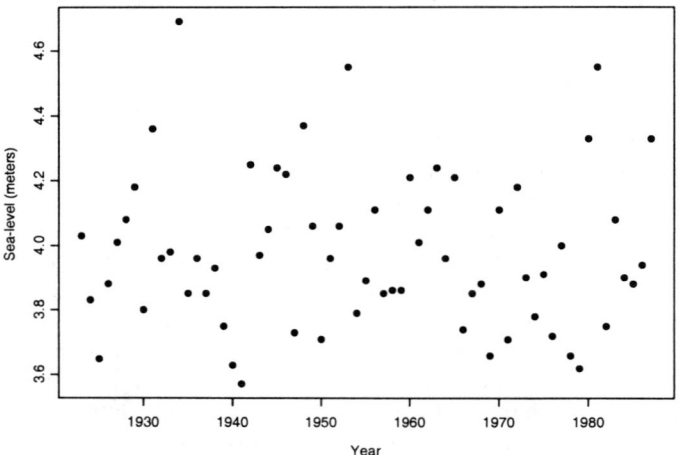

FIGURE 1.1. Annual maximum sea levels at Port Pirie, South Australia.

Example 1.1 Fig. 1.1 shows the annual maximum sea-levels recorded at Port Pirie, a location just north of Adelaide, South Australia, over the period 1923–1987. From such data it may be necessary to obtain an estimate of the maximum sea-level that is likely to occur in the region over the next 100 or 1000 years. This raises an important point – how can we estimate what levels may occur in the next 1000 years without knowing, for example, what climate changes might occur? There is no strong evidence in the figure that the pattern of variation in sea-levels has changed over the observation period, but such stability may not persist in the future. This caveat is important: although extreme value theory has indulged itself with terminology such as the "1000-year return level", corresponding to the level that is expected to be exceeded exactly once in the next 1000 years, this is only meaningful under the assumption of stability (or stationarity) in the prevailing process. It is more realistic to talk in terms of levels that, under current conditions, will occur in a given year with low probability. ▲

Example 1.2 The arguments used for the modeling of extremely large events work equally well for extremely small events, leading to another area of application: reliability modeling. At least conceptually, it is often reasonable to think of a large system as comprised of many smaller components, such that the overall system breaks down if any of the individual components fails. This is the so-called **weakest link principle**, since the strength of the whole system is equal to that of the weakest component. As with maxima, limiting arguments can be adopted to obtain an approximation to the statistical behavior of this weakest link, providing a plausible model for the statistical properties of system failure.

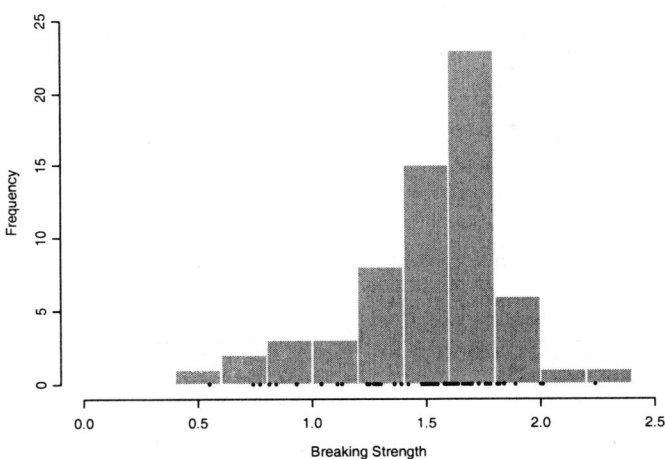

FIGURE 1.2. Histogram of breaking strengths of glass fibers: points indicate actual values.

Fig. 1.2 displays data on breaking strengths of 63 glass fibers of length 1.5 cm, recorded under experimental conditions. The data are reported by Smith & Naylor (1987). The analogy of a weakest link is not perfect in this situation, but it is not unrealistic to consider a glass fiber as a "bundle" of many smaller fibers, such that if any of the small fibers breaks the entire fiber breaks. ▲

Example 1.3 Like in Fig. 1.1, the data in Fig. 1.3 correspond to annual maximum sea-levels, but in this case recorded at Fremantle, near Perth, Western Australia. A careful look at these data suggests that the pattern of variation has not remained constant over the observation period. There is a discernible increase in the data through time, though the increase seems slighter in more recent years.

6   1. Introduction

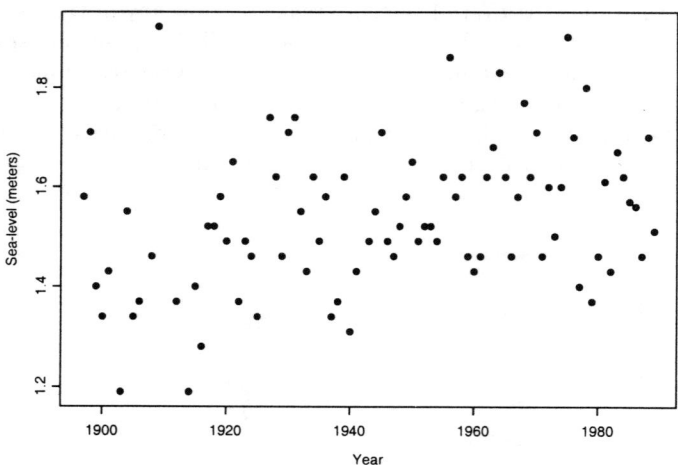

FIGURE 1.3. Annual maximum sea levels at Fremantle, Western Australia.

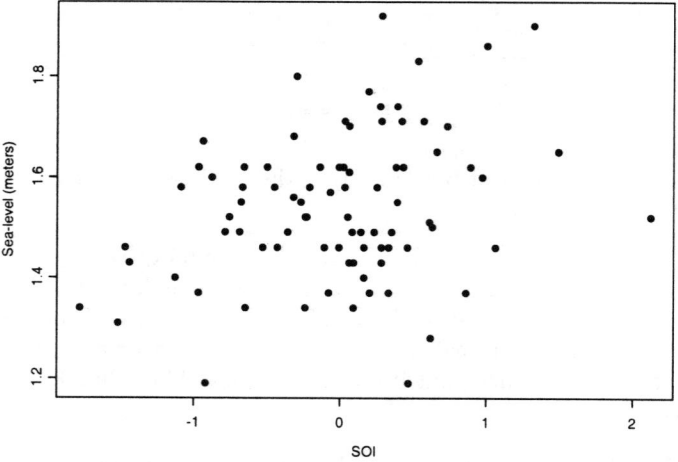

FIGURE 1.4. Annual maximum sea level at Fremantle, Western Australia, versus mean annual value of Southern Oscillation Index.

Identifying such variations in extreme value behavior may be the primary objective of an analysis – just a slight increase in extreme sea-levels could have significant impact on the safety of coastal flood defenses, for example. But even if patterns in variation are not of great interest, to ignore them and to treat the data as if they were time-homogeneous could lead to misleading results and conclusions.

Variations in extreme value behavior can also be caused by other phenomena. For example, pollution levels are likely to be less extreme during periods of high winds, which have a dispersive effect. In the sea-level context, particularly in the southern oceans, extreme sea-levels could be unusually extreme during periods when the El Niño effect is active. As a partial exploration of this phenomenon, Fig. 1.4 shows a plot of the annual maximum sea-level data for Fremantle against the annual mean value of the Southern Oscillation Index (SOI), which is a proxy for meteorological volatility due to effects such as El Niño. It seems from Fig. 1.4 that the annual maximum sea-levels are generally greatest when the value of SOI is high. This may be due to the time trend in the data – annual maximum sea-levels increase with SOI, which itself is increasing through time – but it is also possible that the SOI explains some of the variation in annual maximum sea-levels after allowance for the time variation in the process. Detailed statistical modeling is needed to disentangle these possible effects. ▲

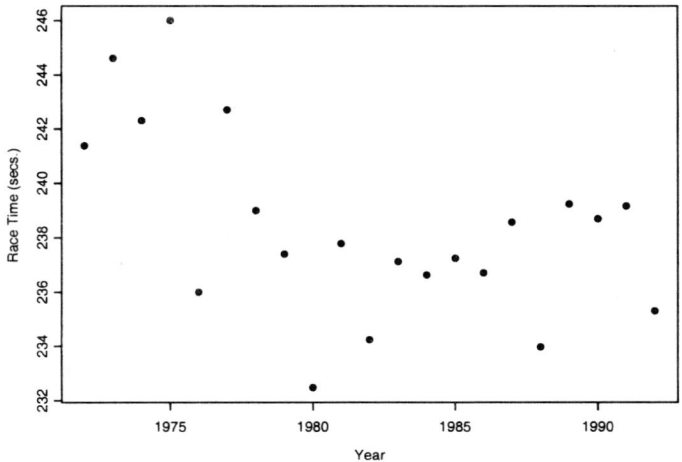

FIGURE 1.5. Fastest annual women's 1500 meters race times.

8   1. Introduction

Example 1.4 A more recreational application of extreme value theory is to the modeling of sports data. Fig. 1.5 shows the fastest annual race times for the women's 1500 meter event over the period 1972–1992, which comprise a subset of the data analyzed using extreme value techniques by Robinson & Tawn (1995). By arguing that the fastest race time in a year corresponds to the fastest race time performed by many athletes within that period, the same argument as applied to the breaking strengths of glass fibers suggests that asymptotic extreme value models might be an appropriate way to model data of this type. Because of improvements in training techniques, race times would be expected to decrease through time, and this is borne out by Fig. 1.5. So, like for the sea-level data of Example 1.3, the model structure should describe not just the pattern of variation of fastest race times within any given year, but also the systematic variation across years. ▲

Example 1.5 As discussed in Section 1.1, it is vital to exploit as much relevant information as is available in an extreme value analysis. A direct approach is to model more of the observed extremes than the annual maxima. For some processes, not just the largest observation in a year, but perhaps the largest 5 or 10 observations, are recorded. These are termed the largest 5 (or 10) order statistics.

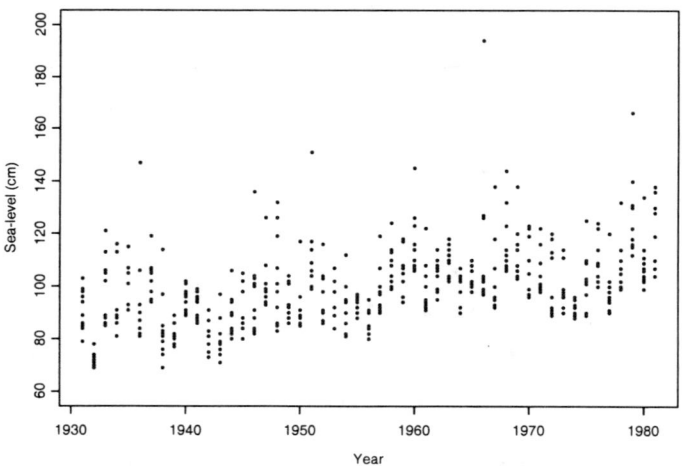

FIGURE 1.6. Largest 10 annual sea-levels in Venice.

As an example, Fig. 1.6 displays the 10 largest sea-levels each year in Venice for the period 1931–1981, except for the year 1935 in which only the 6 largest measurements are available. The data were first studied using contemporary extreme value techniques by Smith (1986). The additional information that is available – relative to the annual maxima only – can be used to improve estimation of the variation within each year, as well as the apparent variation through time. ▲

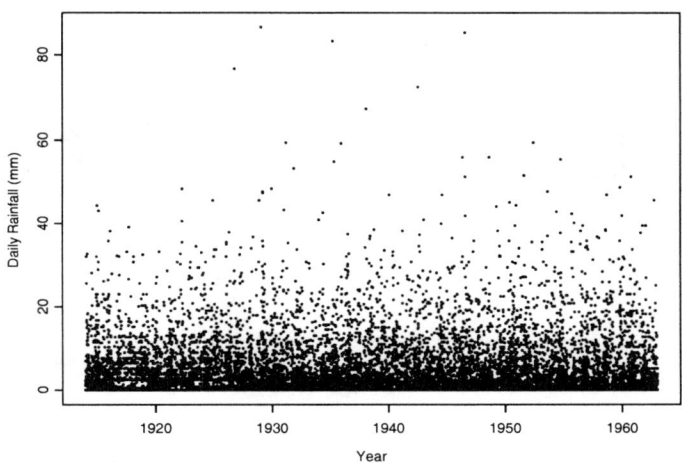

FIGURE 1.7. Daily rainfall accumulations.

Example 1.6 Methods for modeling either block maxima or the largest order statistics within blocks are of historical interest because of the way extreme value theory has developed as a scientific discipline. But if a complete time series of observations is available, then it is almost certainly more efficient to use alternative representations of extremes that enable more of the available information to contribute to the analysis.

Fig. 1.7 shows a time series of daily rainfall accumulations at a location in south-west England recorded over the period 1914–1962. These data form part of a study made by Coles & Tawn (1996b). If the appropriate statistical model for such data were known, the complete dataset could be used to estimate a model which might be extrapolated to high levels of the process. In the absence of such knowledge, we again use an asymptotic model as an approximation. But rather than artificially blocking the data into years, and extracting the maximum from each block, it is more efficient to define an event as being extreme if it falls above some high level, perhaps a daily rainfall of 30 mm in this case. This requires a different model development – extremes are now those observations that exceed a high threshold – so the argument focuses on approximations for high thresholds, rather than long blocks. Efficiency is improved because all observations that are extreme in the sense of exceeding a high threshold can be used in model fitting. ▲

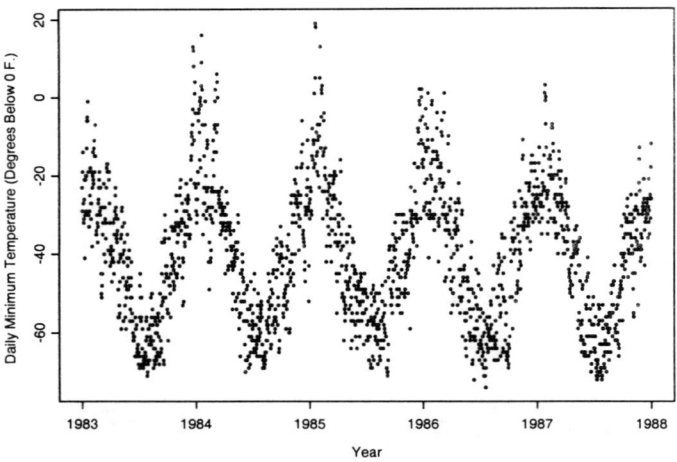

FIGURE 1.8. Negated Wooster daily minimum temperatures.

Example 1.7 A simplifying aspect of the rainfall data example is the absence of any strong pattern of variation, either within a particular year, or from one year to another. Such series are said to be stationary. Though detailed analysis is likely to suggest that such an assumption is not completely accurate for the rainfall data, the near-stationarity makes the modeling of such data relatively straightforward.

Most environmental datasets have a more complex structure than this. In particular, time-dependent variation and short-term clustering are typical phenomena for extreme value data, and it is crucial that both are properly accounted for when making inferences. For example, Fig. 1.8 shows a 5-year series of daily minimum temperatures recorded in Wooster, Ohio. Extremes of a longer version of this series were studied by Smith et al. (1997) and Coles et al. (1994). The data are plotted as degrees Fahrenheit below zero, so that large positive observations correspond to extreme cold conditions. There is a strong annual cycle in the data, so it would be unreasonable to use models that assume a time-constant random variation of the process. In particular, an exceptionally cold winter day has quite different characteristics from an exceptionally cold summer day. A tendency for extreme values to occur close to one another is also apparent in Fig. 1.8. ▲

1.2 Examples   11

Example 1.8 Extreme value techniques are becoming increasingly popular in financial applications. This is not surprising: financial solubility of an investment is likely to be determined by extreme changes in market conditions rather than typical changes. The complex stochastic structure of financial markets does mean, however, that naive application of extreme value techniques can be misleading.

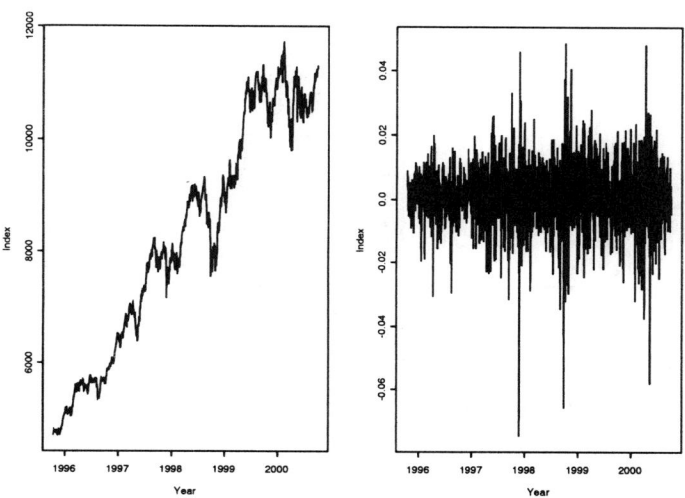

FIGURE 1.9. Left panel: daily closing prices of the Dow Jones Index. Right panel: log-daily returns of the Dow Jones Index.

Fig. 1.9 shows the daily closing prices of the Dow Jones Index over a 5-year period. Evidently, the level of the process has changed dramatically over the observed period, and issues about extremes of daily behavior are swamped by long-term time variation in the series. Like the Wooster temperature data, the process is non-stationary, but now in a way that is not simply explained by trends or seasonal cycles. Many empirical studies on series of this type have indicated that an approximation to stationarity can be obtained by taking logarithms of ratios of successive observations – the so-called log-daily returns. For the Dow Jones Index data this series is also plotted in Fig. 1.9; it suggests a reasonably successful transformation to stationarity. Analysis of the extreme value properties of such transformed series can provide financial analysts with key market information. ▲

Example 1.9 Another way to incorporate extra information in an extreme value analysis is to model more than one series simultaneously. For example, Fig. 1.10 shows the corresponding annual maximum wind speeds over the

12   1. Introduction

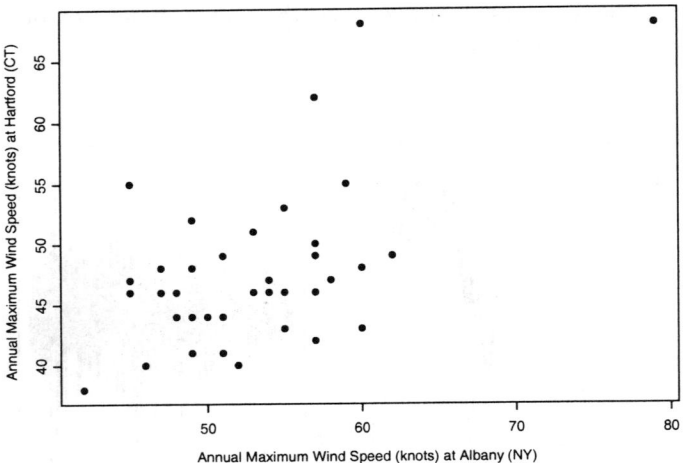

FIGURE 1.10. Annual maximum wind speeds at Albany (NY) and Hartford (CT).

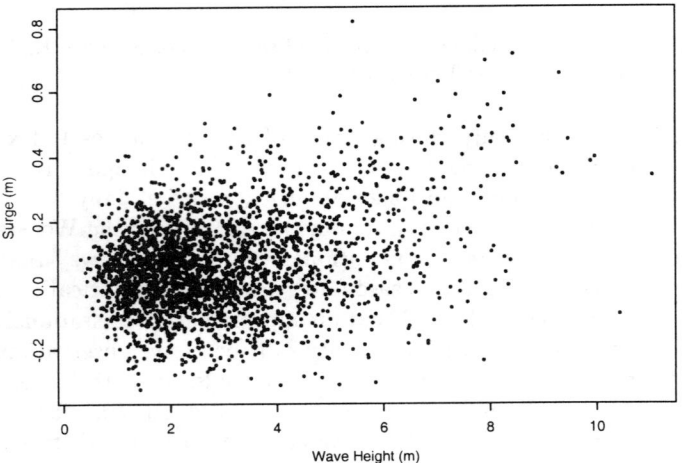

FIGURE 1.11. Concurrent wave and surge heights.

period 1944–1983 at two locations in the United States: Albany, New York and Hartford, Connecticut. From the figure there appears to be a tendency for a high annual maximum wind speed at one location to be associated with a correspondingly high value at the other. That is, the extreme values are dependent, presumably because meteorological events occur on a spatial scale that includes both locations. Because of the dependence, information from either location may be useful in estimating the extreme value behavior at the other location. Furthermore, quantifying the dependence across locations may itself be informative: extreme wind speeds occurring over a large region can have more serious implications for risk assessment and environmental protection than localized extreme events. ▲

Example 1.10 Restriction to annual maximum data is also a wasteful approach to extreme value modeling in a multivariate setting if complete data on each variable are available. For example, Fig. 1.11 shows concurrent measurements of two oceanographic variables – wave and surge height – at a single location off south-west England. The figure suggests a tendency for extremes of one variable to coincide with extremes of the other. Identifying such a phenomenon is likely to be important, as the impact of an event that is simultaneously extreme may be much greater than if extremes of either component occur in isolation. Multivariate extreme value models enable the calculation of the probability of simultaneously extreme events, though this requires an asymptotic approximation for the dependence at extreme levels, as well as the extreme value behavior of each individual series. ▲

Example 1.11 As well as having a complex structure through time, financial series may also be dependent with comparable series. Fig. 1.12 shows series of the log-daily returns of two exchange rates: UK sterling against both the US dollar and the Canadian dollar. Careful inspection of the series suggests that they vary in harmony with each other, a phenomenon that is due to synchronization of the US and Canadian financial markets. The effect is seen more clearly in Fig. 1.13, which shows concurrent values of one series against the other.

Harmonization across financial markets is a major issue for risk analysts, particularly when risk or investment is spread across various commodities within a single portfolio. To understand the overall level of risk entailed by a specific portfolio, questions about the extent of dependence between extremes of a number of series become unavoidable. ▲

1.3 Structure of the Book

The aim of this book is not to give a complete overview of all approaches to extreme value analysis, but to describe and illustrate techniques for a

14   1. Introduction

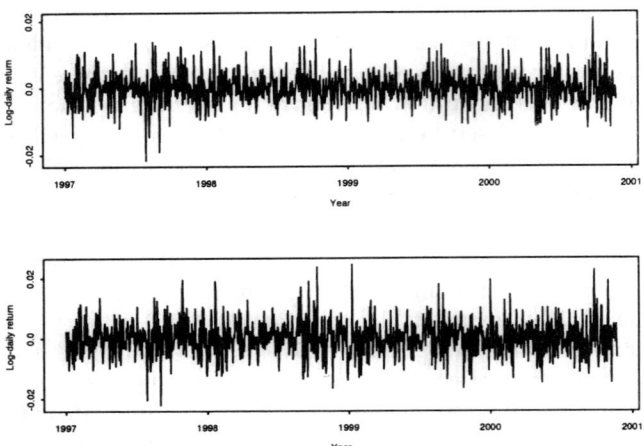

FIGURE 1.12. Log-daily returns of exchange rates. Top panel: UK sterling/US dollar exchange rate. Bottom panel: UK sterling/Canadian dollar exchange rate.

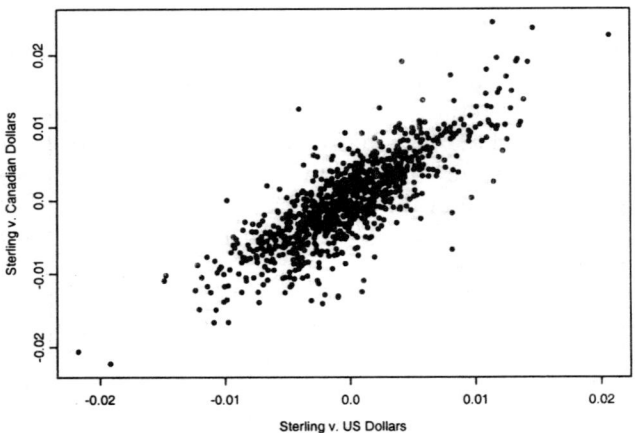

FIGURE 1.13. Concurrent log-daily returns of UK sterling/US dollar exchange rate and UK sterling/Canadian dollar exchange rate.

specific approach that exploits the opportunities made available by contemporary techniques in statistical modeling. A general overview of statistical modeling techniques is described in Chapter 2. This chapter is also not comprehensive, but limited to results and procedures that are required in subsequent chapters. In particular, techniques of modeling via the likelihood function are discussed in some detail. Readers with statistical expertise might prefer to skip this chapter, and refer back to it only when necessary.

Subsequent chapters return to various specific themes of extreme value modeling. In order to keep the mathematical level of the book reasonably elementary, some detail in model development is sacrificed in favor of heuristics. Rather more attention is given to the statistical modeling issues that arise in the implementation of the models, using the examples discussed in Section 1.2 to illustrate the various techniques.

Chapter 3 deals with the classical theory of extremes. Primarily this concerns the development of models for block maxima (or minima) data, of the type discussed in Examples 1.1 and 1.2. The generalization that enables the modeling of the largest order statistics within blocks, as described in the context of the Venice sea-level data in Example 1.5, is also discussed.

Chapter 4 develops threshold excess models, which are appropriate for modeling the extremes of data when a complete series is available, as in Examples 1.6 and 1.7. Again, a heuristic argument is presented to justify the model, with an emphasis on procedures for statistical modeling in practice.

The model development in Chapters 3 and 4 assumes an underlying series of independent and identically distributed random variables. This makes the arguments simpler, but the assumption is unrealistic for most practical applications. Chapters 5 and 6 discuss the modeling of extremes of processes that are more plausible representations for genuine data series. Chapter 5 deals with stationary sequences – series that may be dependent through time, but have a homogeneity of stochastic behavior. In this case, though we give only brief details, broadly applicable models comparable to those of Chapters 3 and 4 are obtained. Chapter 6 deals with non-stationary processes – processes whose stochastic behavior changes through time, perhaps due to trends or seasonality. Several of the examples of Section 1.2 are evidently non-stationary: the sea-level data of Example 1.3 and the athletics data of Example 1.4 have apparent trends, while the temperature data of Example 1.7 display strong seasonality. In such cases, little can be derived in terms of formal probability results, and it is more fruitful to exploit statistical modeling techniques that allow for – and quantify – the non-homogeneity in extremal behavior.

Chapter 7 gives a unifying characterization of the extremes of processes that encompasses each of the models derived in Chapters 3 and 4, and which also provides a more flexible framework for modeling extremes of non-stationary processes like the temperature series of Example 1.7. This characterization is based on the theory of point processes. A brief introduction to this theory is given, though the main emphasis is on practical implementation for the modeling of extremes.

Chapter 8 describes the basic theory of multivariate extremes (cf. Examples 1.9 and 1.10). The development given follows the treatment of univariate extremes: we start with block maxima, generalize to a threshold excess model and describe a point process representation that encompasses each of the other models. We also discuss the issue of asymptotic independence, which is a condition whose theoretical properties have been well understood, but which has only recently been recognized as an important consideration for statistical modeling.

Through Chapters 3 to 8 we focus only on mainstream issues and techniques for modeling extreme values. Inevitably, this means that very many issues which may be important for specific applications are omitted. As a partial compensation for this, Chapter 9 comprises a brief introduction to a number of other topics: Bayesian inference, Markov chain models and spatial extremes.

All of the computations in this book were carried out in the statistical programming language S-PLUS. Except for the specialized techniques required for Chapter 9, functions to carry out the examples discussed throughout the book are available for download over the internet. Details are given in the Appendix, together with a description of the available functions and a worked example.

1.4 Further Reading

Each subsequent chapter contains references to literature that either expands on, or gives examples of, the material developed in that particular chapter. However, there are a number of texts and articles that are more general in their scope. Leadbetter et al. (1983), Galambos (1987) and Resnick (1987) all provide rigorous treatments of the mathematical foundations of extreme value models. Galambos (1995) also gives a brief review of the subject's theoretical foundations.

On the statistical side, the classic work by Gumbel (1958) is relevant for more than just its historical value. More recent works that offer an alternative viewpoint from the present text are provided by Castillo (1988) and Reiss & Thomas (2001). The latter also includes software for carrying out a range of extreme value analyses. Kotz & Nadarajah (2000), like this book, aims to give an elementary survey of extreme value theory and practice. Smith (1991a) gives a brief contemporary overview of statistical techniques for extreme value modeling, from a similar perspective to that used in this book.

A detailed treatment of the role of extreme value theory primarily for insurance and financial applications is given by Embrechts et al. (1998).

There has also been a recent explosion in the number of articles written on extreme value techniques in the financial literature. For example, Diebold et al. (1997), McNeil & Frey (2000) and Longin (2000) give general overviews, while Wiggins (1992), Koedijk & Kool (1992), Broussard & Booth (1998) and Ho et al. (2000) describe specific applications.

Finally, Tiago de Oliveira (1984b) and Galambos et al. (1994) are compendiums of conference proceedings that contain a variety of articles addressing specific theoretical and methodological aspects of extreme value theory.

2
Basics of Statistical Modeling

2.1 Introduction

It is easiest to introduce concepts by way of example. Suppose we are interested in studying variations from day to day in rainfall levels measured at a particular location. The sequence of observed daily rainfall levels constitute the data, denoted $x_1, \ldots x_n$. On any particular day, prior to measurement, the rainfall level is an uncertain quantity: even with sophisticated weather maps, future rainfall levels cannot be predicted exactly. So, the rainfall on day i is a random quantity, X_i. Once measured, the value is known to be x_i. The distinction between lower and upper case letters is that the upper-case X_i represents the random quantity, whose realized value is subsequently measured as the lower-case x_i. Obviously, although X_i is a random quantity, in the sense that until measured it could take a range of different values, some values are more likely than others. Thus, X_i is assumed to have a probability distribution which attaches probabilities to the various values or ranges of values that X_i might take, and values that are more likely have a higher probability than those which are not.

The data, $x_1, \ldots, x_n$, are a complete record of the rainfall pattern that actually occurred. But the role of statistics is not so much to summarize what has already happened, but to infer the characteristics of randomness in the process that generated the data. For example, the mean daily rainfall over the observation period might have been 3 mm, but what could we then conclude about the mean daily rainfall over a much longer period? Maybe 40% of the x_i were zero, corresponding to dry days, but what is the chance that tomorrow will be dry? And if 6 cm was the largest value of the x_i, what conclusions might we draw about the levels of heavy rainfall that can be anticipated in the future? Statistics addresses these questions by regarding the sequence $x_1, \ldots, x_n$ as realizations of the sequence of random variables $X_1, \ldots, X_n$, and by using the data to estimate the probabilistic structure of these random variables.

It is simplest if the probability distribution on each day is identical. Over long periods, seasonal changes in meteorological conditions are likely to cause a change in patterns of variation of rainfall levels, but over short periods an assumption of similar day-to-day behavior might be reasonable. In this case, assuming that each of the observed data $x_1, \ldots, x_n$ derives from the same probability distribution, relatively straightforward techniques of estimation can be applied. The situation is simpler still if it can be assumed that the daily observations are independent, so that variations in rainfall level on any particular day are not influenced by knowledge of the values for any other days. This also may be unrealistic: the chance of a day being free of rain may be substantially greater if the previous few days were dry rather than wet. That is, the probability distribution of the X_i may be altered by knowledge of $x_1, \ldots, x_{i-1}$.

The remainder of this chapter formalizes these ideas and develops suitable techniques of model estimation and validation. These techniques form the inferential methodology that is applied to the extreme value analyses in subsequent chapters.

2.2 Basic Statistical Concepts

2.2.1 Random Variables and Their Distributions

The basic ingredients of a statistical model are the following. First, a random variable X, which represents a quantity whose outcome is uncertain. The set of possible outcomes of X, denoted Ω, is the **sample space**. Second, a **probability distribution**, which assigns probabilities to events associated with X. There are two distinct possibilities to consider. A random variable X is said to be a **discrete random variable** if its sample space is discrete: $\Omega = \{0, 1, 2, \ldots\}$, for example. In this case, the probability distribution is determined by the **probability mass function**, which takes the form

$$f(x) = \Pr\{X = x\},$$

for each value of x in Ω. Thus, $f(x)$ is the probability that the random variable X takes the value x. For example, if $X =$ "number of consecutive dry days", $f(2)$ would be the probability of 2 consecutive dry days.

Most of the random variables to which extreme value techniques are applied are **continuous random variables**: they have a sample space,

Ω, that is continuous. For example, sea-levels, wind speeds, race times and breaking strengths all take values on a continuous scale. Because of the continuity it is not possible to assign probabilities to all possible values of the random variable in a meaningful way. Loosely speaking, there are simply too many possible values on a continuous scale. Instead, probability distributions can be specified by their **probability distribution function**, defined as

$$F(x) = \Pr\{X \leq x\}, \qquad (2.1)$$

for each x in Ω. For the usual axioms of probability to be satisfied, F must be a non-decreasing function of x, such that $F(x_-) = 0$ and $F(x_+) = 1$, where x_- and x_+ are the lower and upper limits of Ω, respectively. Though it no longer makes sense to talk about probabilities of individual values of x, we can calculate from (2.1) the probabilities of X falling within intervals as

$$\Pr\{a \leq X \leq b\} = F(b) - F(a).$$

If the distribution function F is differentiable, it is also useful to define the **probability density function** of X as

$$f(x) = \frac{dF}{dx},$$

in which case

$$F(x) = \int_{-\infty}^{x} f(u) du$$

and

$$\Pr\{a \leq X \leq b\} = \int_{a}^{b} f(u) du.$$

It is often convenient to summarize a probability distribution by one or two statistics that characterize its main features. The most common are the expectation and variance. In the case of a continuous random variable[1] with probability density function f, the **expectation** is

$$E(X) = \int_{\Omega} x f(x) dx, \qquad (2.2)$$

and the **variance** is

$$\text{Var}(X) = \int_{\Omega} \{x - E(X)\}^2 f(x) dx. \qquad (2.3)$$

Expectation provides a measure of location, or average value, of the distribution, while the variance measures the dispersion or spread of the distribution. The **standard deviation** is defined as the square root of the variance, providing a measure of variability in the same units as X.

---

[1] For discrete variables similar definitions can be made, replacing density functions with mass functions and integration with summation.

2.2.2 Families of Models

In both discrete and continuous cases there are standard families of probability distributions. A simple example in the discrete case is the binomial distribution, which arises in the following way. Suppose we look at a sequence of n independent trials, in each of which the outcome is either a "success" or a "failure", with a common success probability of p in each trial. Denoting by X the total number of successes in the n trials, from elementary probability arguments the probability mass function of X is

$$f(x) = \binom{n}{x} p^x (1-p)^{n-x}, \quad x \in \Omega = \{0, 1, 2, \ldots, n\},$$

where

$$\binom{n}{x} = \frac{n!}{x!(n-x)!}$$

is the number of different ways of choosing x distinct objects from n. In this case, X is said to have a **binomial distribution** with parameters n and p, denoted $X \sim \text{Bin}(n, p)$.

Another important example is the **Poisson distribution**, corresponding to a random variable having probability mass function

$$f(x) = \frac{e^{-\lambda} \lambda^x}{x!}, \quad x \in \Omega = \{0, 1, 2, \ldots\},$$

where the parameter $\lambda > 0$. The Poisson distribution is fundamental as a model for the occurrence of randomly occurring events in time: if events occur randomly in time at an average rate of λ, and the occurrence of one event neither encourages nor inhibits the occurrence of another, then X, the number of events arising in a unit time interval, has a Poisson distribution with parameter λ.

A standard example in the continuous case is the normal distribution. A random variable X is said to have a **normal distribution** with parameters μ and σ, denoted $X \sim \text{N}(\mu, \sigma^2)$, if its probability density function has the form

$$f(x) = \frac{1}{\sqrt{(2\pi\sigma^2)}} \exp\left\{-\frac{(x-\mu)^2}{2\sigma^2}\right\}, \quad x \in \mathbb{R},$$

where μ and $\sigma > 0$ are fixed parameters that equate to the expectation and standard deviation of X. If $X \sim \text{N}(\mu, \sigma^2)$, it can easily be shown that

$$Z = \frac{X - \mu}{\sigma} \sim \text{N}(0, 1).$$

The standardized variable Z is said to follow the **standard normal distribution**. The distribution function of the standard normal distribution, conventionally denoted by $\Phi(z)$, is available from standard statistical tables or software packages. This enables probability calculations on any normally distributed random variable. For example, if $X \sim N(\mu, \sigma^2)$,

$$\begin{aligned} \Pr\{a \leq X \leq b\} &= \Pr\left\{\frac{a-\mu}{\sigma} \leq Z \leq \frac{b-\mu}{\sigma}\right\} \\ &= \Phi\left(\frac{b-\mu}{\sigma}\right) - \Phi\left(\frac{a-\mu}{\sigma}\right). \end{aligned}$$

A related distribution is the chi-squared distribution. If $Z_1, \ldots, Z_k$ are independent standard normal random variables, the variable

$$X = Z_1^2 + \ldots + Z_k^2$$

is said to have a **chi-squared distribution with k degrees of freedom**, denoted $X \sim \chi_k^2$. Many standard test statistics are found to have a distribution that is, at least approximately, a chi-squared distribution. The chi-squared distribution function also requires numerical evaluation from standard tables or software packages.

2.3 Multivariate Distributions

A multivariate random variable is a vector of random variables

$$\boldsymbol{X} = \begin{bmatrix} X_1 \\ \vdots \\ X_k \end{bmatrix}.$$

Notation is made more compact by writing $\boldsymbol{X} = (X_1, \ldots, X_k)^T$, where the operator ^{T} denotes transpose. Each of the components X_i is a random variable in its own right, but specification of the properties of $\boldsymbol{X}$ as a whole requires information about the influence of every variable on each of the others. For example, the X_i might represent different oceanographic variables, all of which are large during storms. Knowledge that one component is large therefore increases the probability that the other components are large.

Generalizing the single variable case, the **joint distribution function** of $\boldsymbol{X}$ is defined by

$$F(\boldsymbol{x}) = \Pr\{X_1 \leq x_1, \ldots, X_k \leq x_k\},$$

where $\boldsymbol{x} = (x_1, \ldots, x_k)$. When the X_i are continuous random variables, and provided it exists, the **joint density function** is given by

$$f(\boldsymbol{x}) = \frac{\partial^k F}{\partial x_1 \cdots \partial x_k}.$$

In this case

$$F(\boldsymbol{x}) = \int_{-\infty}^{x_1} \cdots \int_{-\infty}^{x_k} f(u_1, \ldots, u_k) du_k \ldots du_1,$$

while for any set $\mathcal{A} \subset \mathbb{R}^k$,

$$\Pr\{\boldsymbol{X} \in \mathcal{A}\} = \int \cdots \int_{\mathcal{A}} f(\boldsymbol{u}) d\boldsymbol{u}.$$

The probability density functions of each of the individual X_i, termed **marginal density functions**, are obtained by integrating out the other components. For example,

$$f_{X_1}(x_1) = \int_{-\infty}^{\infty} \cdots \int_{-\infty}^{\infty} f(x_1, u_2, \ldots, u_k) du_k \ldots du_2$$

is the marginal probability density function of the component X_1. Similarly,

$$f_{X_1,X_2}(x_1, x_2) = \int_{-\infty}^{\infty} \cdots \int_{-\infty}^{\infty} f(x_1, x_2, u_3, \ldots, u_k) du_k \ldots du_3$$

is the joint marginal density function of (X_1, X_2).

In the special situation where the outcome of one random variable has no effect on the probability distribution of another, the variables are said to be independent. Formally, the variables X_1 and X_2 are **independent** if their joint density function factorizes, i.e.

$$f_{X_1,X_2}(x_1, x_2) = f_{X_1}(x_1) f_{X_2}(x_2).$$

This definition extends in the obvious way to an arbitrary set of random variables: the variables $X_1, \ldots, X_k$ are **mutually independent** if

$$f_{X_1,\ldots,X_k}(x_1, \ldots, x_k) = \prod_{i=1}^{k} f_{X_i}(x_i). \tag{2.4}$$

More generally, the influence of one random variable on the probability structure of another is characterized by the **conditional density function**:

$$f_{X_1|X_2}(x_1 \mid X_2 = x_2) = \frac{f_{X_1,X_2}(x_1, x_2)}{f_{X_2}(x_2)}.$$

In the case of independent random variables,

$$f_{X_1|X_2}(x_1 \mid X_2 = x_2) = f_{X_1}(x_1),$$

but generally the conditional density function depends also on the value of x_2.

Definitions (2.2) and (2.3) apply to each margin in turn to give measures of the location and dispersion of each marginal component. It is also useful, however, to summarize the extent of dependence between components; that is, the extent to which the components increase or decrease in harmony. The usual summaries are pairwise. The **covariance** of the variables X and Y, having joint density function $f_{X,Y}$, is defined by

$$\text{Cov}(X,Y) = \int_{-\infty}^{\infty} \int_{-\infty}^{\infty} \{x - \text{E}(X)\}\{y - \text{E}(Y)\} f_{X,Y}(x,y) dx dy.$$

The covariance is often re-scaled to obtain a measure on a fixed interval. This leads to the **correlation coefficient**, defined by

$$\text{Corr}(X,Y) = \frac{\text{Cov}(X,Y)}{\sqrt{\text{Var}(X)\text{Var}(Y)}}.$$

The correlation coefficient has a similar interpretation to the covariance, but is such that $-1 \leq \text{Corr}(X,Y) \leq 1$. For independent random variables the correlation is zero. The converse, however, is false, as the correlation is a measure only of the extent to which variables are linearly associated. Consequently, variables may have zero correlation if their association is non-linear.

For a general random vector $\boldsymbol{X} = (X_1, \ldots, X_k)^T$, it is usual to pack together all of the information on variances and covariances between each pair of variables into a matrix, the **variance-covariance matrix**, defined as

$$\Sigma = \begin{bmatrix} \sigma_{1,1} & \cdots & & \sigma_{1,k} \\ \vdots & \ddots & \sigma_{i,j} & \vdots \\ & \sigma_{j,i} & \ddots & \\ \sigma_{k,1} & \cdots & & \sigma_{k,k} \end{bmatrix}$$

where $\sigma_{i,i} = \text{Var}(X_i)$ and $\sigma_{i,j} = \text{Cov}(X_i, X_j)$ for $i \neq j$.

Like in the univariate case, there are standard families of probability distributions for random vectors. In particular, the multivariate analogue of the normal distribution is the multivariate normal distribution: the random variable $\boldsymbol{X} = (X_1, \ldots X_k)^T$ is said to follow a **multivariate normal distribution** with mean vector $\boldsymbol{\mu} = (\mu_1, \ldots, \mu_k)^T$ and variance-covariance matrix Σ, denoted $\boldsymbol{X} \sim \text{MVN}_k(\boldsymbol{\mu}, \Sigma)$, if its joint density function has the form

$$f_{\boldsymbol{X}}(\boldsymbol{x}) = \frac{1}{(2\pi)^{k/2} |\Sigma|^{1/2}} \exp\left\{-\frac{1}{2}(\boldsymbol{x} - \boldsymbol{\mu})^T \Sigma^{-1} (\boldsymbol{x} - \boldsymbol{\mu})\right\}, \quad \boldsymbol{x} \in \mathbb{R}^k,$$

where $|\Sigma|$ is the determinant of Σ. This definition implies that each of the marginal distributions is normal and that the complete joint distribution is determined once the marginal means and the variance-covariance matrix are specified.

2.4 Random Processes

2.4.1 Stationary Processes

A sequence of random variables $X_1, X_2, \ldots$ is said to be a (discrete time) **random process**.[2] The simplest example of a random process is a sequence of independent and identically distributed random variables, though this model is usually too simple as a description of real-life phenomena. First, data series often display dependence through time – in particular, values of a process are often dependent on the recent history of the process. Second, their random behavior is often observed to vary over time – seasonal variations are intrinsic to many natural processes, for example. These two issues are usually addressed separately, and it is convenient first to study processes that may exhibit dependence, but whose stochastic behavior is homogeneous through time. This leads to the notion of stationarity.

Definition 2.1 A random process $X_1, X_2, \ldots$ is said to be **stationary** if, given any set of integers $\{i_1, \ldots, i_k\}$ and any integer m, the joint distributions of $(X_{i_1}, \ldots, X_{i_k})$ and $(X_{i_1+m}, \ldots, X_{i_k+m})$ are identical. △

Stationarity implies that, given any subset of variables, the joint distribution of the same subset viewed m time points later remains unchanged. Unlike an independent series, stationarity does not preclude X_i being dependent on previous values, although X_{i+m} must have the same dependence on its previous values. On the other hand, trends, seasonality and other deterministic cycles are excluded by an assumption of stationarity.

2.4.2 Markov Chains

For some applications it is necessary to give a more detailed prescription of the stochastic behavior of a random process. For a stationary sequence of independent variables, it is enough just to specify the marginal distribution. More generally, it is necessary to specify the distribution of an arbitrary term in the sequence, X_i, conditional on all the previous values, $X_1, \ldots, X_{i-1}$. Excluding independence, the simplest class is when this conditional distribution depends only on the most recent observation. That is, whilst the future evolution of the process may depend on its current value, once that value is known the earlier history is irrelevant. Such a series is said to be a first-order Markov chain. We give the definition for a process whose values occur on a continuous space; an analogous definition holds for processes taking values on a discrete space, with probability mass functions replacing density functions.

---

[2] Continuous time random processes can also be defined.

Definition 2.2 A random process $X_1, X_2, \ldots$ is a **first-order Markov chain** if, for every $i = 2, 3, \ldots$, the conditional density function satisfies

$$f(x_i \mid x_{i-1}, \ldots, x_1) = f(x_i \mid x_{i-1}).$$

△

Markov chain models are widely used in statistical modeling, partly because they provide the simplest generalization of independent processes, partly because they are easy to estimate and partly because their properties are well-understood. They can also be generalized to allow dependence on the most recent k observations rather than just the most recent – this is a kth-order Markov chain. Because of the dependence of consecutive values in a Markov chain, the distribution of any future value X_{i+m} is likely to depend on the current value X_i. However, for a wide class of Markov chains the dependence diminishes as m becomes large. In other words, a term in the sequence is influenced by the recent history of the series, but much less by its distant past. In this case the chain is said to have a **stationary distribution**, which is the distribution of X_n as $n \to \infty$, the point being that the eventual stochastic properties of the process do not depend on the initial condition of the chain.

2.5 Limit Laws

It is often difficult to perform exact calculations with probability distributions. This might be because the distribution is unknown, or simply because the analytical or computational burden is high. In these situations it may be possible to approximate the true distribution by a simpler distribution obtained by a limiting argument. This requires a definition of convergence of random variables. There are several possibilities, but the most useful for our purposes is convergence in distribution.

Definition 2.3 A sequence of random variables $X_1, X_2, \ldots$, having distribution functions $F_1, F_2, \ldots$ respectively, is said to **converge in distribution** to the random variable X, having distribution function F, denoted $X_n \xrightarrow{d} X$, if

$$F_n(x) \to F(x) \quad \text{as} \quad n \to \infty$$

for all continuity points x of F. △

For statistical applications, the utility of establishing a limit distribution F for a sequence of random variables $X_1, X_2 \ldots$ is usually to justify the use of F as an approximation to the distribution of X_n for large n.

The most celebrated limit law in statistics is the **central limit theorem**, stated here in its simplest form.

Theorem 2.1 Let $X_1, X_2, \ldots$ be a sequence of independent and identically distributed random variables with mean μ and finite, positive variance σ^2. Then, defining

$$\bar{X}_n = \frac{X_1 + \cdots + X_n}{n},$$

$$\frac{\sqrt{n}(\bar{X}_n - \mu)}{\sigma} \xrightarrow{d} Z \qquad (2.5)$$

as $n \to \infty$, where $Z \sim N(0, 1)$. □

The central limit theorem is generally used in statistical applications by interpreting (2.5) as an approximation for the distribution of the sample mean $\bar{X}_n$ for large n. That is,

$$\bar{X}_n \overset{\cdot}{\sim} N(\mu, \sigma^2/n)$$

for large n, where the notation $\overset{\cdot}{\sim}$ denotes "is approximately distributed as". What makes the central limit theorem remarkable, and so useful for application, is that the approximating distribution of the sample mean is normal regardless of the parent population of the X_i. Analogous arguments are used in subsequent chapters to obtain approximating distributions for sample extremes.

2.6 Parametric Modeling

2.6.1 The Parametric Framework

As we have discussed, a common objective in statistical modeling is to use sample information to make inferences on the probability structure of the population from which the data arose. In the simplest case, the data $x_1, \ldots, x_n$ are assumed to be independent realizations from the population distribution. Inference then amounts to estimation of this distribution, for which there are two distinct approaches: parametric or nonparametric. We concentrate on the parametric approach. The first step is to adopt a family of models within which the true distribution of the data is assumed to lie. This might be based on physical grounds: for example, idealized radioactive counts are bound to follow a Poisson distribution. More often, a model is chosen on empirical grounds, using exploratory techniques to ascertain families of models that look broadly consistent with the available data. Another alternative is the use of limit laws as approximations. We have already discussed this in the context of using the normal distribution as an approximation for sample means, and the approach will also be central to our development of extreme value models.

In the subsequent discussion we restrict discussion to the case of a continuous random variable whose probability density function exists, though the arguments apply more widely. We also suppose that the data $x_1, \ldots, x_n$ comprise independent realizations of a random variable X whose probability density function belongs to a known family of probability distributions with density functions $\mathcal{F} = \{f(x;\theta) : \theta \in \Theta\}$. We denote[3] the true value of the parameter θ by θ_0. Inference is therefore reduced to estimation of the true parameter value θ_0 from within the parameter space Θ. The parameter θ may be a scalar, such as $\theta = p$ in the binomial family, or it may represent a vector of parameters, such as $\theta = (\mu, \sigma)$ in the normal family.

2.6.2 Principles of Estimation

Assume for the moment that the parameter θ in $\mathcal{F}$ is scalar rather than vector. A function of random variables that is used to estimate the true parameter value θ_0 is called an **estimator**; the particular value of the estimator for an observed set of data is the **estimate**. Since the data are outcomes of random variables, repeats of the experiment would generate different data and hence a different estimate. Thus, randomness in the sampling process induces randomness in the estimator. The probability distribution induced in an estimator is said to be its **sampling distribution**.

It is desirable that estimates are close to the parameter value they are estimating. This leads to two definitions. The **bias** of an estimator $\hat{\theta}_0$ of θ_0 is defined by

$$\text{Bias}(\hat{\theta}_0) = E(\hat{\theta}_0) - \theta_0,$$

and the **mean-square error** by

$$\text{MSE}(\hat{\theta}_0) = \text{E}\{(\hat{\theta}_0 - \theta_0)^2\}.$$

An estimator whose bias is zero is said to be **unbiased**; this corresponds to an estimator whose value, on average, is the true parameter value. It is usually difficult to arrange for estimators to be unbiased, but anticipated that the bias is small. A more common criterion for estimator assessment is that its MSE should be small. Since the MSE measures variation of the estimator around the true parameter value, low MSE implies that in any particular sample the estimate is likely to be close to the true parameter value.

As the sampling distribution determines the variability of an estimator, simple summaries of the distribution lead to measures of accuracy. The standard deviation of the sampling distribution of $\hat{\theta}_0$ is called the **standard error**, denoted $\text{SE}(\hat{\theta}_0)$. Usually, an approximation of $\text{SE}(\hat{\theta}_0)$ can be calculated using the observed sample. Since this measures the extent of variability in the estimator, and provided the bias of the estimator is neg-

---

[3] In subsequent sections, we drop the distinction and use θ to denote both an arbitrary parameter value and the true parameter value.

ligible, $\text{SE}(\hat{\theta}_0)$ is implicitly a measure of how precise the estimator is: the smaller the standard error, the greater the precision.

Quantifying the precision of an estimator can usually be made more explicit by calculating a confidence interval. This is especially easy if a pivot is available. A **pivot** is a function of $\hat{\theta}_0$ and θ_0 whose distribution does not depend on θ_0. If $\phi = g(\hat{\theta}_0, \theta_0)$ is a pivot, since its sampling distribution does not depend on unknown parameters, for any value of $0 < \alpha < 1$ it is possible to find limits ϕ_u and ϕ_l such that

$$\Pr\{\phi_l \leq \phi \leq \phi_u\} = 1 - \alpha.$$

This can be rearranged to give

$$\Pr\{\theta_l \leq \theta_0 \leq \theta_u\} = 1 - \alpha,$$

where θ_l and θ_u are functions of ϕ_l, ϕ_u and $\hat{\theta}_0$. The interval $[\theta_l, \theta_u]$ is said to be a $(1 - \alpha)$ **confidence interval** for θ_0.

The rationale for a confidence interval is that it expresses a range of values for which we can be "confident" that the true parameter value lies. The choice of α is arbitrary: small values give high confidence but wide intervals; large values give small intervals but low confidence. This implies a trade-off between the width of the interval and the degree of confidence that the interval contains the true parameter value. Commonly used values are $\alpha = 0.05, 0.01$ and 0.001, corresponding to $95\%, 99\%$ and 99.9% confidence intervals respectively.

As an example, suppose we want to estimate a population mean μ on the basis of independent realizations $x_1, \ldots x_n$ drawn from the population. Assume also that the variance of the population, σ^2, is unknown. A natural estimator of μ is the sample mean

$$\bar{X} = n^{-1}(X_1 + \cdots + X_n),$$

which is easily checked to be unbiased for μ. Also, $\text{Var}(\bar{X}) = \sigma^2/n$, so that $\text{SE}(\bar{X}) = \sigma/\sqrt{n}$. Approximating the unknown value of σ with the sample standard deviation s leads to $\text{SE}(\bar{X}) \approx s/\sqrt{n}$.

Approximate confidence intervals can also be obtained since, by the central limit theorem,

$$\bar{X} - \mu \overset{.}{\sim} N(0, \sigma^2/n),$$

so that $\bar{X} - \mu$ is a pivot. By standard manipulation,

$$\Pr\{-z_{\frac{\alpha}{2}}\sigma/\sqrt{n} \leq \bar{X} - \mu \leq z_{\frac{\alpha}{2}}\sigma/\sqrt{n}\} = 1 - \alpha, \tag{2.6}$$

where $z_{\frac{\alpha}{2}}$ is the $(1 - \alpha/2)$ quantile of the standard normal distribution. Rearranging (2.6) gives

$$\Pr\{\bar{X} - z_{\frac{\alpha}{2}}\sigma/\sqrt{n} \leq \mu \leq \bar{X} + z_{\frac{\alpha}{2}}\sigma/\sqrt{n}\} = 1 - \alpha,$$

so that
$$[\bar{X} - z_{\frac{\alpha}{2}}\sigma/\sqrt{n}, \bar{X} + z_{\frac{\alpha}{2}}\sigma/\sqrt{n}]$$
is an approximate $(1-\alpha)$ confidence interval for μ. Provided the sample size is reasonably large, this approximation is not adversely affected by replacing the unknown σ by the sample estimate s, leading finally to the confidence interval
$$[\bar{X} - z_{\frac{\alpha}{2}}s/\sqrt{n}, \bar{X} + z_{\frac{\alpha}{2}}s/\sqrt{n}].$$

2.6.3 Maximum Likelihood Estimation

A general and flexible method of estimation of the unknown parameter θ_0 within a family $\mathcal{F}$ is maximum likelihood. Each value of $\theta \in \Theta$ defines a model in $\mathcal{F}$ that attaches (potentially) different probabilities (or probability densities) to the observed data. The probability of the observed data as a function of θ is called the likelihood function. Values of θ that have high likelihood correspond to models which give high probability to the observed data. The principle of maximum likelihood estimation is to adopt the model with greatest likelihood, since of all the models under consideration, this is the one that assigns highest probability to the observed data.

In greater detail, referring back to the situation in which $x_1, \ldots, x_n$ are independent realizations of a random variable having probability density function $f(x; \theta_0)$, the **likelihood function** is

$$L(\theta) = \prod_{i=1}^{n} f(x_i; \theta). \tag{2.7}$$

The factorization in (2.7) is due to (2.4) for independent observations. It is often more convenient to take logarithms and work with the **log-likelihood function**

$$\ell(\theta) = \log L(\theta) = \sum_{i=1}^{n} \log f(x_i; \theta). \tag{2.8}$$

Both (2.7) and (2.8) generalize in the obvious way to the situation where the X_i are independent, but not necessarily with identical distributions. In this case, denoting the density function of X_i by $f_i(x_i; \theta)$, we obtain

$$L(\theta) = \prod_{i=1}^{n} f_i(x_i; \theta),$$

and

$$\ell(\theta) = \sum_{i=1}^{n} \log f_i(x_i; \theta).$$

More generally still, if $\mathcal{F} = \{f(\boldsymbol{x};\theta) : \theta \in \Theta\}$ denotes a family of joint probability density functions for a set of (not necessarily independent) observations $\boldsymbol{x} = (x_1, \ldots, x_n)$, then the likelihood is

$$L(\theta) = f(\boldsymbol{x};\theta),$$

regarded as a function of θ with $\boldsymbol{x}$ fixed at the observed value.

The **maximum likelihood estimator** $\hat{\theta}_0$ of θ_0 is defined as the value of θ that maximizes the appropriate likelihood function. Since the logarithm function is monotonic, the log-likelihood takes its maximum at the same point as the likelihood function, so that the maximum likelihood estimator also maximizes the corresponding log-likelihood function.

For some examples it is possible to obtain the maximum likelihood estimator explicitly, usually by differentiating the log-likelihood and equating to zero. For example, if $X_1 \ldots X_n$ are independent Poi(λ) variables, it is easy to check that $\hat{\lambda} = \bar{x}$, the sample mean. In the corresponding normal example, $(\hat{\mu}, \hat{\sigma}) = (\bar{x}, s)$, where s is the sample standard deviation. In more complicated examples it is usually necessary to apply numerical techniques to maximize the log-likelihood.

2.6.4 Approximate Normality of the Maximum Likelihood Estimator

A substantial benefit of adopting maximum likelihood as a principle for parameter estimation is that standard and widely applicable approximations are available for a number of useful sampling distributions. These lead to approximations for standard errors and confidence intervals. There are several useful results. The framework is as above: $x_1, \ldots, x_n$ are independent realizations of a random variable X having distribution $F \in \mathcal{F}$. The family $\mathcal{F}$ is indexed by a d-dimensional parameter θ and the true distribution F has $\theta = \theta_0$. The maximum likelihood estimate of θ_0 is denoted $\hat{\theta}_0$.

Strictly, each of the results is an asymptotic limit law obtained as the sample size n increases to infinity. They are also valid only under regularity conditions. We will assume these conditions to be valid and give the results as approximations whose accuracy improves as n increases.

Theorem 2.2 Let $x_1, \ldots, x_n$ be independent realizations from a distribution within a parametric family $\mathcal{F}$, and let $\ell(\cdot)$ and $\hat{\theta}_0$ denote respectively the log-likelihood function and the maximum likelihood estimator of the d-dimensional model parameter θ_0. Then, under suitable regularity conditions, for large n

$$\hat{\theta}_0 \stackrel{.}{\sim} \text{MVN}_d(\theta_0, I_E(\theta_0)^{-1}), \tag{2.9}$$

where

$$I_E(\theta) = \begin{bmatrix} e_{1,1}(\theta) & \cdots & & e_{1,d}(\theta) \\ \vdots & \ddots & e_{i,j}(\theta) & \vdots \\ & e_{j,i}(\theta) & \ddots & \\ e_{d,1}(\theta) & \cdots & & e_{d,d}(\theta) \end{bmatrix},$$

with

$$e_{i,j}(\theta) = E\left\{-\frac{\partial^2}{\partial\theta_i \partial\theta_j}\ell(\theta)\right\}.$$

□

The matrix $I_E(\theta)$, which measures the expected curvature of the log-likelihood surface, is usually referred to as the **expected information matrix**.

Theorem 2.2 can be used to obtain approximate confidence intervals for individual components of $\theta_0 = (\theta_1, \ldots, \theta_d)$. Denoting an arbitrary term in the inverse of $I_E(\theta_0)$ by $\psi_{i,j}$, it follows from the properties of the multivariate normal distribution that, for large n,

$$\hat{\theta}_i \overset{.}{\sim} N(\theta_i, \psi_{i,i}).$$

Hence, if $\psi_{i,i}$ were known, an approximate $(1-\alpha)$ confidence interval for θ_i would be

$$\hat{\theta}_i \pm z_{\frac{\alpha}{2}} \sqrt{\psi_{i,i}}, \tag{2.10}$$

where $z_{\frac{\alpha}{2}}$ is the $(1 - \alpha/2)$ quantile of the standard normal distribution. Since the true value of θ_0 is generally unknown, it is usual to approximate the terms of I_E with those of the **observed information matrix**, defined by

$$I_O(\theta) = \begin{bmatrix} -\frac{\partial^2}{\partial\theta_1^2}\ell(\theta) & \cdots & & -\frac{\partial^2}{\partial\theta_1\partial\theta_d}\ell(\theta) \\ \vdots & \ddots & -\frac{\partial^2}{\partial\theta_i\partial\theta_j}\ell(\theta) & \vdots \\ & -\frac{\partial^2}{\partial\theta_j\partial\theta_i}\ell(\theta) & \ddots & \\ -\frac{\partial^2}{\partial\theta_d\partial\theta_1}\ell(\theta) & \cdots & & -\frac{\partial^2}{\partial\theta_d^2}\ell(\theta) \end{bmatrix}$$

and evaluated at $\theta = \hat{\theta}$. Denoting the terms of the inverse of this matrix by $\tilde{\psi}_{i,j}$, it follows that an approximate $(1-\alpha)$ confidence interval for θ_i is

$$\hat{\theta}_i \pm z_{\frac{\alpha}{2}} \sqrt{\tilde{\psi}_{i,i}}.$$

Despite the additional approximation, such intervals are often more accurate than those obtained in (2.10).

Although a parametric family $\mathcal{F}$ may be indexed by a parameter θ, of which θ_0 represents the true value, it may not be θ_0 that is of particular interest. Instead, it may be some function $\phi_0 = g(\theta_0)$ that we wish to estimate, where ϕ_0 may have a different dimension to θ_0. We restrict attention to the situation where ϕ_0 is a scalar function of θ_0. This is often useful in extreme value modeling, where θ_0 is the parameter vector of a distribution representing extreme value behavior, but it is the probability of some extreme event – which is a function of θ_0 – that is needed. The following two results enable maximum likelihood inferences on θ_0 to be transformed to give corresponding inferences on ϕ_0.

Theorem 2.3 If $\hat{\theta}_0$ is the maximum likelihood estimate of θ_0, and $\phi = g(\theta)$ is a scalar function, then the maximum likelihood estimate of ϕ_0 is given by $\hat{\phi}_0 = g(\hat{\theta}_0)$. □

This result means that, once the maximum likelihood estimate of θ_0 has been calculated, the maximum likelihood estimate of any function of θ_0 is obtained by simple substitution.

Theorem 2.4 Let $\hat{\theta}_0$ be the large-sample maximum likelihood estimator of the d-dimensional parameter θ_0 with approximate variance-covariance matrix V_θ. Then if $\phi = g(\theta)$ is a scalar function, the maximum likelihood estimator of $\phi_0 = g(\theta_0)$ satisfies

$$\hat{\phi}_0 \stackrel{.}{\sim} N(\phi_0, V_\phi),$$

where

$$V_\phi = \nabla \phi^T V_\theta \nabla \phi,$$

with

$$\nabla \phi = \left[\frac{\partial \phi}{\partial \theta_1}, \ldots, \frac{\partial \phi}{\partial \theta_d} \right]^T$$

evaluated at $\hat{\theta}_0$. □

Theorem 2.4 is usually referred to as the **delta method**. In the same way that the approximate normality of $\hat{\theta}_0$ can be used to obtain confidence intervals for the individual components of θ_0, the delta method enables the approximate normality of $\hat{\phi}_0$ to be used to obtain confidence intervals for ϕ_0.

2.6.5 Approximate Inference Using the Deviance Function

An alternative method for quantifying the uncertainty in the maximum likelihood estimator is based on the **deviance function**, defined by

$$D(\theta) = 2\{\ell(\hat{\theta}_0) - \ell(\theta)\}. \qquad (2.11)$$

Values of θ with a small deviance correspond to models with a high likelihood, so a natural criterion for deriving confidence regions is to specify as a confidence region
$$C = \{\theta : D(\theta) \le c\}$$
for some choice of c. Ideally, we would like to choose c in such a way that the corresponding region C has a pre-specified probability, $(1-\alpha)$ say, of containing the true parameter θ_0. In general this is not possible, as it would require knowledge of the population distribution. Even if this distribution were known, the exact calculations needed to determine the distribution of $D(\theta)$ are unlikely to be tractable. These difficulties are usually resolved by using an approximation to the sampling distribution that is valid for large sample sizes.

Theorem 2.5 Let $x_1, \ldots, x_n$ be independent realizations from a distribution within a parametric family $\mathcal{F}$, and let $\hat{\theta}_0$ denote the maximum likelihood estimator of the d-dimensional model parameter θ_0. Then for large n, under suitable regularity conditions, the deviance function (2.11) satisfies
$$D(\theta_0) \overset{\cdot}{\sim} \chi_d^2.$$

$\square$

It follows from Theorem 2.5 that an approximate $(1-\alpha)$ confidence region for θ_0 is given by
$$C_\alpha = \{\theta : D(\theta) \le c_\alpha\},$$
where c_α is the $(1-\alpha)$ quantile of the χ_d^2 distribution. This approximation is usually more accurate than that based on the asymptotic normality of the maximum likelihood estimator, though the computational burden is greater.

2.6.6 Inference Using the Profile Likelihood Function

We described in Section 2.6.4 one method for making inferences on a particular component θ_i of a parameter vector θ. An alternative, and usually more accurate, method is based on profile likelihood. The log-likelihood for θ can be formally written as $\ell(\theta_i, \theta_{-i})$, where θ_{-i} denotes all components of θ excluding θ_i. The **profile log-likelihood** for θ_i is defined as
$$\ell_p(\theta_i) = \max_{\theta_{-i}} \ell(\theta_i, \theta_{-i}).$$

That is, for each value of θ_i, the profile log-likelihood is the maximized log-likelihood with respect to all other components of θ. In other words, $\ell_p(\theta_i)$ is the profile of the log-likelihood surface viewed from the θ_i axis.

2.6 Parametric Modeling

This definition generalizes to the situation where θ can be partitioned into two components, $(\theta^{(1)}, \theta^{(2)})$, of which $\theta^{(1)}$ is the k-dimensional vector of interest and $\theta^{(2)}$ corresponds to the remaining $(d-k)$ components. The profile log-likelihood for $\theta^{(1)}$ is now defined as

$$\ell_p(\theta^{(1)}) = \max_{\theta^{(2)}} \ell(\theta^{(1)}, \theta^{(2)}).$$

If $k = 1$ this reduces to the previous definition.

The following result, which generalizes Theorem 2.5, leads to a procedure for approximate inferences on the maximum likelihood estimator of $\theta^{(1)}$.

Theorem 2.6 Let $x_1, \ldots, x_n$ be independent realizations from a distribution within a parametric family $\mathcal{F}$, and let $\hat{\theta}_0$ denote the maximum likelihood estimator of the d-dimensional model parameter $\theta_0 = (\theta^{(1)}, \theta^{(2)})$, where $\theta^{(1)}$ is a k-dimensional subset of θ_0. Then, under suitable regularity conditions, for large n

$$D_p(\theta^{(1)}) = 2\{\ell(\hat{\theta}_0) - \ell_p(\theta^{(1)})\} \stackrel{.}{\sim} \chi_k^2.$$

□

Theorem 2.6 is frequently used in two different situations. First, for a single component θ_i, $C_\alpha = \{\theta_i : D_p(\theta_i) \leq c_\alpha\}$ is a $(1-\alpha)$ confidence interval, where c_α is the $(1-\alpha)$ quantile of the χ_1^2 distribution. This yields an alternative, and usually more accurate, method to that based on Theorem 2.2. The second application is to model selection. Suppose that $\mathcal{M}_1$ is a model with parameter vector θ, and model $\mathcal{M}_0$ is the subset of model $\mathcal{M}_1$ obtained by constraining k of the components of θ to be, say, zero. Hence, θ can be partitioned as $\theta = (\theta^{(1)}, \theta^{(2)})$, where the first component, of dimension k, is zero in model $\mathcal{M}_0$. Now, let $\ell_1(\mathcal{M}_1)$ be the maximized log-likelihood for model $\mathcal{M}_1$, let $\ell_0(\mathcal{M}_0)$ be the maximized log-likelihood for model $\mathcal{M}_0$, and define

$$D = 2\{\ell_1(\mathcal{M}_1) - \ell_0(\mathcal{M}_0)\}$$

to be the **deviance statistic**. By Theorem 2.6, $C_\alpha = \{\theta^{(1)} : D_p(\theta^{(1)}) \leq c_\alpha\}$ comprises a $(1-\alpha)$ confidence region for the true value of $\theta^{(1)}$, where D_p is the profile deviance and c_α is the $(1-\alpha)$ quantile of the χ_k^2 distribution. Hence, to check whether $\mathcal{M}_0$ is a plausible reduction of model $\mathcal{M}_1$, it is sufficient to check whether 0 lies in C_α, which is equivalent to checking if $D < c_\alpha$. This is termed a **likelihood ratio test**, summarized as follows.

Theorem 2.7 Suppose $\mathcal{M}_0$ with parameter $\theta^{(2)}$ is the sub-model of $\mathcal{M}_1$ with parameter $\theta_0 = (\theta^{(1)}, \theta^{(2)})$ under the constraint that the k-dimensional sub-vector $\theta^{(1)} = \mathbf{0}$. Let $\ell_0(\mathcal{M}_0)$ and $\ell_1(\mathcal{M}_1)$ be the maximized values of the log-likelihood for models $\mathcal{M}_0$ and $\mathcal{M}_1$ respectively. A test of the validity of model $\mathcal{M}_0$ relative to $\mathcal{M}_1$ at the α level of significance is to reject $\mathcal{M}_0$ in favor of $\mathcal{M}_1$ if $D = 2\{\ell_1(\mathcal{M}_1) - \ell_0(\mathcal{M}_0)\} > c_\alpha$, where c_α is the $(1-\alpha)$ quantile of the χ_k^2 distribution. □

Finally, we remark that, under additional regularity, each of the large sample approximations described in this section is valid when $x_1, \ldots, x_n$ are independent but non-identically distributed realizations from a family indexed by a parameter θ. For example, in a classical regression model, $X_i \sim \mathcal{D}(\alpha + \beta w_i)$ for $i = 1, \ldots, n$, where $\mathcal{D}(\theta)$ denotes a distribution with parameter θ and $w_1, \ldots, w_n$ are known constants. Although each of the X_i has a different distribution, the maximum likelihood estimator of (α, β) still satisfies the large sample properties stated in Theorems 2.2–2.7.

2.6.7 Model Diagnostics

The reason for fitting a statistical model to data is to make conclusions about some aspect of the population from which the data were drawn. Such conclusions can be sensitive to the accuracy of the fitted model, so it is necessary to check that the model fits well. The main issue concerns the ability of the model to describe variations in the wider population, but this is usually unachievable unless there are additional sources of data against which the model can be judged. Consequently, the only option that is normally available is to judge the accuracy of a model in terms of its agreement with the data that were actually used to estimate it.

Suppose data $x_1, \ldots, x_n$ are independent realizations from a common population with unknown distribution function F. An estimate of F, say $\hat{F}$, has been obtained, perhaps by maximum likelihood, and we want to assess the plausibility that the x_i are a random sample from $\hat{F}$. First, a model-free estimate of F can be obtained empirically from the data. Let $x_{(1)}, \ldots, x_{(n)}$ denote the ordered sample, so that $x_{(1)} \leq x_{(2)} \leq \cdots \leq x_{(n)}$. For any one of the $x_{(i)}$, exactly i of the n observations have a value less than or equal to $x_{(i)}$, so an empirical estimate of the probability of an observation being less than or equal to $x_{(i)}$ is $\tilde{F}(x_{(i)}) = i/n$. A slight adjustment to $\tilde{F}(x_{(i)}) = i/(n+1)$ is usually made to avoid having $\tilde{F}(x_{(n)}) = 1$. This leads to the following definition.

Definition 2.4 Given an ordered sample of independent observations

$$x_{(1)} \leq x_{(2)} \leq \cdots \leq x_{(n)}$$

from a population with distribution function F, the **empirical distribution function** is defined by

$$\tilde{F}(x) = \frac{i}{n+1} \quad \text{for } x_{(i)} \leq x < x_{(i+1)}.$$

△

Since $\tilde{F}$ is an estimate of the true probability distribution F, it should be in reasonable agreement with the candidate model, $\hat{F}$, provided $\hat{F}$ is an adequate estimate of F. Various goodness-of-fit procedures are based on comparisons of $\tilde{F}$ and $\hat{F}$. Two graphical techniques, in particular, are commonly used.

Definition 2.5 Given an ordered sample of independent observations

$$x_{(1)} \leq x_{(2)} \leq \cdots \leq x_{(n)}$$

from a population with estimated distribution function $\hat{F}$, a **probability plot** consists of the points

$$\left\{ \left(\hat{F}(x_{(i)}), \frac{i}{n+1} \right) : i = 1, \ldots, n \right\}.$$

△

If $\hat{F}$ is a reasonable model for the population distribution, the points of the probability plot should lie close to the unit diagonal. Substantial departures from linearity provide evidence of a failure in $\hat{F}$ as a model for the data.

Definition 2.6 Given an ordered sample of independent observations

$$x_{(1)} \leq x_{(2)} \leq \cdots \leq x_{(n)}$$

from a population with estimated distribution function $\hat{F}$, a **quantile plot** consists of the points

$$\left\{ \left(\hat{F}^{-1}\left(\frac{i}{n+1}\right), x_{(i)} \right) : i = 1, \ldots, n \right\}.$$

△

The name "quantile plot" derives from the fact that the quantities $x_{(i)}$ and $\hat{F}^{-1}(i/(n+1))$ each provide estimates of the $i/(n+1)$ quantile of the distribution F. If $\hat{F}$ is a reasonable estimate of F, then the quantile plot should also consist of points close to the unit diagonal.

The probability plot and the quantile plot contain the same information expressed on a different scale. However, the perception gained on different scales can be important, so what looks like a reasonable fit on one scale, may look poor on the other.

38   2. Basics of Statistical Modeling

2.7 Example

We conclude this chapter with an example that illustrates most of the techniques discussed in earlier sections. The model falls outside of the class of extreme value models that form the core of this book, though there are connections with the threshold excess models discussed in Chapter 4.

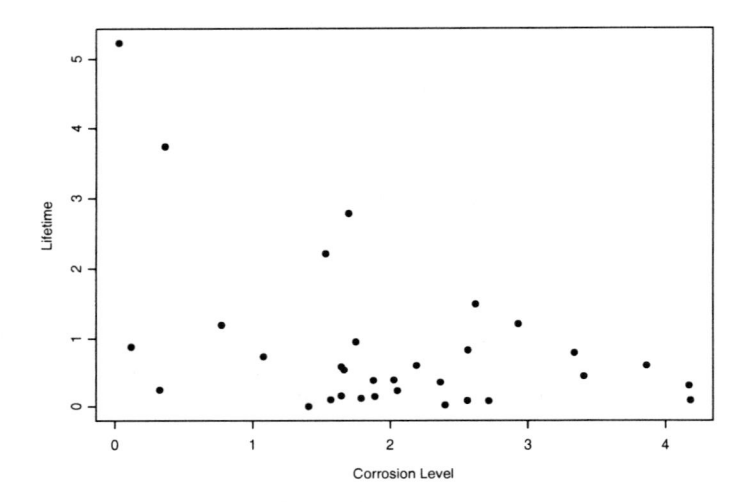

FIGURE 2.1. Engine component failure times against corrosion level.

The data shown in Fig. 2.1 represent simulated time to failure of a sample of 32 engine components with different levels of corrosion. Each component has been assigned a measure of corrosion, and the aim of the analysis is to ascertain how failure time is affected by the corrosion level.

We denote the data by the pairs $\{(w_1, t_1), \ldots, (w_n, t_n)\}$, where t_i is the failure time and w_i is the corrosion level for engine i. In the present analysis we regard the w_i as fixed and the t_i as the realizations of random variables whose dependence on the w_i is to be explored. Since the failure times are non-negative, it is unlikely that the normal distribution would provide a good model. As an alternative, we consider models based on the exponential distribution. A random variable T is said to follow an exponential distribution with parameter λ, denoted $T \sim \text{Exp}(\lambda)$, if its probability density function has the form

$$f(t) = \lambda e^{-\lambda t}, \quad t > 0, \tag{2.12}$$

where $\lambda > 0$. It is easily verified that $\text{E}(T) = 1/\lambda$, so that λ is the reciprocal mean.

Allowing for the possible effect of the covariate w requires a model for its influence on t. Because of the relationship between λ and the distribution mean, this is equivalent to specifying a relationship between the mean lifetime and w. The basic idea of parametric modeling is to specify a flexible family of models for this relationship, ensuring that the family includes models having the broad pattern that the data demonstrate. The parameters of the model can then be estimated by maximum likelihood. In this particular example, judging from Fig. 2.1, the mean lifetime should be permitted to decrease monotonically with increasing values of w, whilst respecting a constraint to maintain positivity. One possible model is

$$T \sim \text{Exp}(\lambda),$$

where

$$\lambda = aw^b \tag{2.13}$$

for parameters a and b. Equivalent to (2.13), $\text{E}(T) = a^{-1}w^{-b}$, so that mean lifetime is modeled as varying exponentially with w at a rate determined by the parameter b; unless $b = 0$, in which case $\text{E}(T) = a^{-1}$ for each engine.

The likelihood for the model is easily evaluated from (2.12) as

$$L(a,b) = \prod_{i=1}^{n} \left\{ aw_i^b e^{-aw_i^b t_i} \right\},$$

leading to the log-likelihood

$$\ell(a,b) = n \log a + b \sum_{i=1}^{n} \log w_i - a \sum_{i=1}^{n} w_i^b t_i. \tag{2.14}$$

The maximum likelihood estimate is found by maximizing this expression with respect to a and b. In principle, this can be done by solving the equations

$$\frac{\partial \ell}{\partial a} = \frac{n}{a} - \sum_{i=1}^{n} w_i^b t_i = 0,$$

$$\frac{\partial \ell}{\partial b} = \sum_{i=1}^{n} \log w_i - a \sum_{i=1}^{n} w_i^b t_i \log w_i = 0,$$

but since the equations have no analytical solution, numerical techniques are required. In that case, direct numerical maximization of ℓ (or minimization of $-\ell$) in (2.14) is more common, using algorithms routinely available in standard software packages.

Substituting the engine lifetime data, maximization of (2.14) leads to the estimates

$$\hat{a} = 1.133 \quad \text{and} \quad \hat{b} = 0.479,$$

with a maximized log-likelihood of -21.71. The corresponding mean failure time curve,
$$E(T) = 1.133^{-1} \times w^{-0.479},$$
is shown relative to the data in Fig. 2.2. The estimated curve shows a strong variation of mean failure time with the covariate w and seems also to give a reasonable match to the pattern in the observed data.

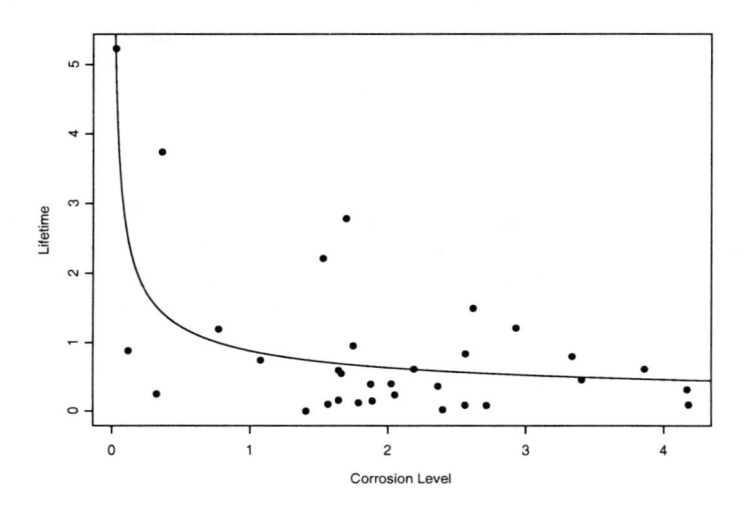

FIGURE 2.2. Engine component failure times against corrosion level. Solid curve shows estimated mean component lifetime as a function of corrosion level.

The observed information matrix in this example is easily calculated as
$$\begin{bmatrix} -\frac{\partial^2 \ell}{\partial q^2} & -\frac{\partial^2 \ell}{\partial a \partial b} \\ -\frac{\partial^2 \ell}{\partial a \partial b} & -\frac{\partial^2 \ell}{\partial b^2} \end{bmatrix} = \begin{bmatrix} na^{-2} & \sum w_i^b t_i \log w_i \\ \sum w_i^b t_i \log w_i & a \sum w_i^b t_i (\log w_i)^2 \end{bmatrix}.$$

As discussed above, it is more convenient and often more accurate to work instead with the observed information matrix. For reference, the expected information can also be evaluated for this model: since $E(T_i) = a^{-1} w_i^{-b}$, we obtain
$$I_E(a,b) = \begin{bmatrix} na^{-2} & a^{-1} \sum \log w_i \\ a^{-1} \sum \log w_i & \sum (\log w_i)^2 \end{bmatrix}.$$

Substitution of the maximum likelihood estimates into the observed information matrix, followed by matrix inversion, leads to the estimated variance-covariance matrix
$$V = \begin{bmatrix} 0.04682 & -0.01442 \\ -0.01442 & 0.03104 \end{bmatrix}.$$

Taking square roots of the diagonal terms, we obtain the standard errors 0.216 and 0.176 for $\hat{a}$ and $\hat{b}$, respectively. Approximate confidence intervals follow. For example, an approximate 95% confidence interval for b is $0.479 \pm 1.96 \times 0.176 = [0.134, 0.824]$. The fact that this interval excludes 0 provides evidence that $b \neq 0$. Formally, the possibility that $b = 0$ is rejected at the 5% level of significance, so the data provide reasonably strong support for a non-degenerate relationship between failure time and corrosion level.

Confidence intervals can also be obtained for other quantities by the delta method. For example, it may be necessary to estimate the mean failure time for an engine component whose corrosion level is $w = w_0$ for some fixed value of w_0. In this case the parameter of interest is $\phi = E(T) = a^{-1} w_0^{-b}$. By the invariance property of maximum likelihood,

$$\hat{\phi} = \hat{a}^{-1} w_0^{-\hat{b}},$$

while by the delta method,

$$\mathrm{Var}(\hat{\phi}) \approx \nabla \phi^T V \nabla \phi, \tag{2.15}$$

where

$$\nabla \phi^T = \left[\frac{\partial \phi}{\partial a}, \frac{\partial \phi}{\partial b} \right] = \left[-a^{-2} w_0^{-b}, -a^{-1} w_0^{-b} \log w_0 \right], \tag{2.16}$$

evaluated at $(\hat{a}, \hat{b})$. For example, an engine with a corrosion level of $w_0 = 3$ has $\hat{\phi} = 1.133 \times 3^{-0.479} = 0.669$, and substitution into (2.15) and (2.16) gives $\mathrm{Var}(\hat{\phi}) = 0.0125$. Hence, a 95% confidence interval for the mean failure time of such an engine is $0.669 \pm 1.96 \times \sqrt{0.0125} = [0.450, 0.889]$.

Greater accuracy in the calculation of confidence intervals is obtained by working with the profile likelihood. In this particular example the profile likelihood for b can be obtained explicitly. Treating b as fixed, the log-likelihood (2.14), regarded as a function of a, is maximized by solving

$$\frac{\partial \ell}{\partial a} = \frac{n}{a} - \sum_{i=1}^{n} w_i^b t_i = 0,$$

leading to

$$\hat{a}_b = \frac{n}{\sum w_i^b t_i}.$$

Hence, the profile likelihood for b is obtained by substitution of this expression into (2.14), giving

$$\ell_p(b) = n \log \hat{a}_b + b \sum_{i=1}^{n} \log w_i - \hat{a}_b \sum_{i=1}^{n} w_i^b t_i.$$

For the data of this example, a plot of the log-likelihood is shown in Fig. 2.3. Based on Theorem 2.6, a 95% confidence interval for b is obtained by drawing a line at a height of $0.5 \times c_{1,0.05}$ below the maximum of this graph, where $c_{1,0.05}$ is the 95% quantile of a χ_1^2 distribution, and reading off the points of intersection. This leads to a 95% confidence interval for b of $[0.183, 0.879]$. Compared with the previous interval of $[0.134, 0.824]$, the profile likelihood interval is similar in width, but is shifted to the right, corresponding to the skewness observed in Fig. 2.3.

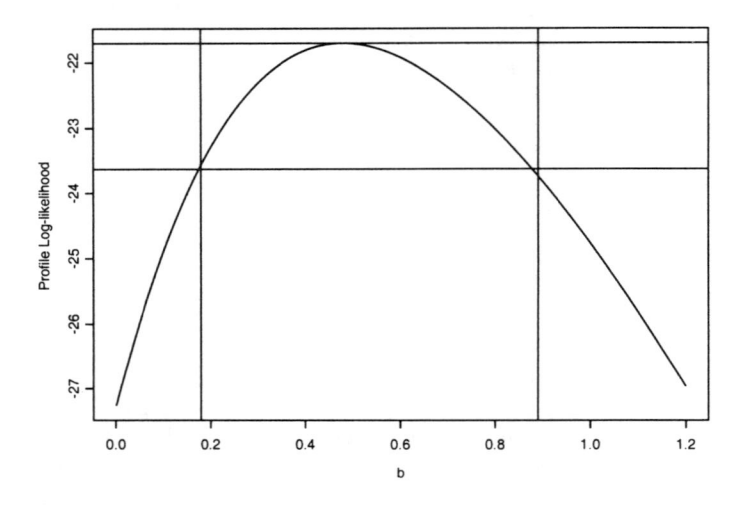

FIGURE 2.3. Profile log-likelihood for b in the engine component failure time example.

As discussed in Section 2.6.6, if a comparison of nested models is required, Theorem 2.6 can be applied without the necessity of producing the entire profile likelihood curve. In this particular example we may be interested in comparing the model (2.13), which we now call $\mathcal{M}_1$, with a simplified model, $\mathcal{M}_0$, in which it is assumed that $T_i \sim \text{Exp}(a)$ for all engines. Thus, model $\mathcal{M}_0$ is a sub-model of $\mathcal{M}_1$ with the constraint that $b = 0$. Model $\mathcal{M}_0$ is of particular interest since it corresponds to an assumption that the lifetime distribution is unaffected by the corrosion level. We have already established that the maximum value of the log-likelihood for model $\mathcal{M}_1$ is -21.71. Model $\mathcal{M}_0$ corresponds to a homogeneous exponential model, for which the log-likelihood is

$$\ell(a) = n \log a - a \sum_{i=1}^{n} t_i. \qquad (2.17)$$

Naturally, this is the same as (2.14) with $b = 0$. Maximizing (2.17) leads to $\hat{a} = n / \sum t_i = 1.159$ for the given data. Substitution into (2.17) then gives a maximized log-likelihood for model $\mathcal{M}_0$ of -27.29. Hence, the deviance statistic for comparing these two models is

$$D = 2\{-21.71 - (-27.29)\} = 11.16.$$

Using the likelihood ratio test (Theorem 2.7), this value is highly significant compared with a χ_1^2 distribution, and therefore provides strong evidence in favor of model $\mathcal{M}_1$, supporting the effect of corrosion level on engine lifetimes. This procedure is operationally equivalent to checking whether or not 0 lies in the profile likelihood interval for b, but is achieved without having to calculate the interval.

Finally, the conclusions reached are dependent on the validity of the assumed model. This is not so straightforward to check because the T_i have non-identical distributions. However, if we assume the fitted model

$$T_i \sim \text{Exp}(\hat{a} w_i^{\hat{b}})$$

to be accurate, then the standardized variables

$$\tilde{T}_i = \hat{a} w_i^{\hat{b}} T_i$$

are such that $\tilde{T}_i \sim \text{Exp}(1)$, using standard properties of the exponential distribution. Hence, we can calculate the values of the standardized variables on the basis of the fitted model, and use probability and quantile plots to compare these against an exponential distribution with parameter 1. With the $\tilde{T}_i$ assumed to be increasing order, a probability plot consists of the pairs

$$\left\{ \left(i/(n+1), 1 - e^{-\tilde{t}_i} \right) ; \; i = 1, \ldots, n \right\},$$

while a quantile plot comprises the pairs

$$\left\{ \left(-\log(1 - i/(n+1)), \tilde{t}_i \right) ; \; i = 1, \ldots, n \right\}.$$

The plots for the engine component failure time data are shown respectively in Figs. 2.4 and 2.5. In both cases the points are sufficiently close to linearity to lend support to the fitted model.

2.8 Further Reading

There are many textbooks that describe the basics of statistical inference and modeling. For theoretical aspects the books by Casella & Berger (2001), Silvey (1970) and Azzalini (1996) are all reasonably elementary. A more advanced text is the classic Cox & Hinkley (1974). On the modeling side, Venables & Ripley (1997) has the added advantage that it also includes an introduction to the statistical language S-PLUS, which is used for the extreme value modeling in subsequent chapters. Grimmett & Stirzaker (1992) provide an elementary account of the probabilistic theory of random processes, including a detailed study of Markov chains.

44   2. Basics of Statistical Modeling

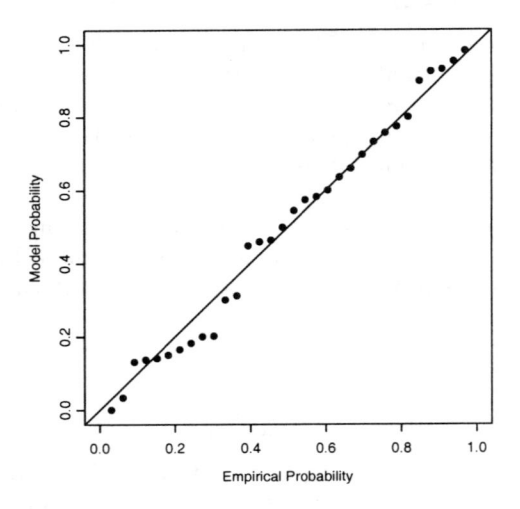

FIGURE 2.4. Probability plot for fitted model in the engine component failure time example.

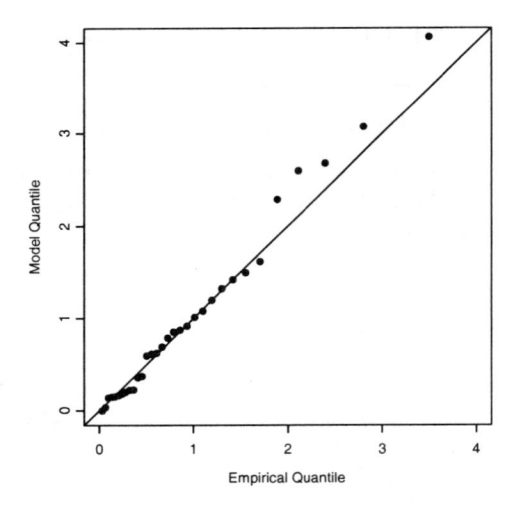

FIGURE 2.5. Quantile plot for fitted model in the engine component failure time example.

3
Classical Extreme Value Theory and Models

3.1 Asymptotic Models

3.1.1 Model Formulation

In this chapter we develop the model which represents the cornerstone of extreme value theory. The model focuses on the statistical behavior of

$$M_n = \max\{X_1, \ldots, X_n\},$$

where $X_1, \ldots, X_n$, is a sequence of independent random variables having a common distribution function F. In applications, the X_i usually represent values of a process measured on a regular time-scale – perhaps hourly measurements of sea-level, or daily mean temperatures – so that M_n represents the maximum of the process over n time units of observation. If n is the number of observations in a year, then M_n corresponds to the annual maximum.

In theory the distribution of M_n can be derived exactly for all values of n:

$$\begin{aligned}
\Pr\{M_n \leq z\} &= \Pr\{X_1 \leq z, \ldots, X_n \leq z\} \\
&= \Pr\{X_1 \leq z\} \times \cdots \times \Pr\{X_n \leq z\} \\
&= \{F(z)\}^n.
\end{aligned} \quad (3.1)$$

However, this is not immediately helpful in practice, since the distribution function F is unknown. One possibility is to use standard statistical

46   3. Classical Extreme Value Theory and Models

techniques to estimate F from observed data, and then to substitute this estimate into (3.1). Unfortunately, very small discrepancies in the estimate of F can lead to substantial discrepancies for F^n.

An alternative approach is to accept that F is unknown, and to look for approximate families of models for F^n, which can be estimated on the basis of the extreme data only. This is similar to the usual practice of approximating the distribution of sample means by the normal distribution, as justified by the central limit theorem. The arguments in this chapter are essentially an extreme value analog of the central limit theory.

We proceed by looking at the behavior of F^n as $n \to \infty$. But this alone is not enough: for any $z < z_+$, where z_+ is the upper end-point of F,[1] $F^n(z) \to 0$ as $n \to \infty$, so that the distribution of M_n degenerates to a point mass on z_+. This difficulty is avoided by allowing a linear renormalization of the variable M_n:

$$M_n^* = \frac{M_n - b_n}{a_n},$$

for sequences of constants $\{a_n > 0\}$ and $\{b_n\}$. Appropriate choices of the $\{a_n\}$ and $\{b_n\}$ stabilize the location and scale of M_n^* as n increases, avoiding the difficulties that arise with the variable M_n. We therefore seek limit distributions for M_n^*, with appropriate choices of $\{a_n\}$ and $\{b_n\}$, rather than M_n.

3.1.2   Extremal Types Theorem

The entire range of possible limit distributions for M_n^* is given by Theorem 3.1, the extremal types theorem.

Theorem 3.1 If there exist sequences of constants $\{a_n > 0\}$ and $\{b_n\}$ such that

$$\Pr\{(M_n - b_n)/a_n \leq z\} \to G(z) \quad \text{as } n \to \infty,$$

where G is a non-degenerate distribution function, then G belongs to one of the following families:

$$\mathrm{I}: G(z) = \exp\left\{-\exp\left[-\left(\frac{z-b}{a}\right)\right]\right\}, \quad -\infty < z < \infty;$$

$$\mathrm{II}: G(z) = \begin{cases} 0, & z \leq b, \\ \exp\left\{-\left(\frac{z-b}{a}\right)^{-\alpha}\right\}, & z > b; \end{cases}$$

$$\mathrm{III}: G(z) = \begin{cases} \exp\left\{-\left[-\left(\frac{z-b}{a}\right)^{\alpha}\right]\right\}, & z < b, \\ 1, & z \geq b, \end{cases}$$

for parameters $a > 0, b$ and, in the case of families II and III, $\alpha > 0$.   □

---

[1]z_+ is the smallest value of z such that $F(z) = 1$.

In words, Theorem 3.1 states that the rescaled sample maxima $(M_n - b_n)/a_n$ converge in distribution to a variable having a distribution within one of the families labeled I, II and III. Collectively, these three classes of distribution are termed the **extreme value distributions**, with types I, II and III widely known as the **Gumbel**, **Fréchet** and **Weibull** families respectively. Each family has a location and scale parameter, b and a respectively; additionally, the Fréchet and Weibull families have a shape parameter α.

Theorem 3.1 implies that, when M_n can be stabilized with suitable sequences $\{a_n\}$ and $\{b_n\}$, the corresponding normalized variable M_n^* has a limiting distribution that must be one of the three types of extreme value distribution. The remarkable feature of this result is that the three types of extreme value distributions are the only possible limits for the distributions of the M_n^*, regardless of the distribution F for the population. It is in this sense that the theorem provides an extreme value analog of the central limit theorem.

3.1.3 The Generalized Extreme Value Distribution

The three types of limits that arise in Theorem 3.1 have distinct forms of behavior, corresponding to the different forms of tail behavior for the distribution function F of the X_i. This can be made precise by considering the behavior of the limit distribution G at z_+, its upper end-point. For the Weibull distribution z_+ is finite, while for both the Fréchet and Gumbel distributions $z_+ = \infty$. However, the density of G decays exponentially for the Gumbel distribution and polynomially for the Fréchet distribution, corresponding to relatively different rates of decay in the tail of F. It follows that in applications the three different families give quite different representations of extreme value behavior. In early applications of extreme value theory, it was usual to adopt one of the three families, and then to estimate the relevant parameters of that distribution. But there are two weaknesses: first, a technique is required to choose which of the three families is most appropriate for the data at hand; second, once such a decision is made, subsequent inferences presume this choice to be correct, and do not allow for the uncertainty such a selection involves, even though this uncertainty may be substantial.

A better analysis is offered by a reformulation of the models in Theorem 3.1. It is straightforward to check that the Gumbel, Fréchet and Weibull families can be combined into a single family of models having distribution functions of the form

$$G(z) = \exp\left\{-\left[1 + \xi\left(\frac{z-\mu}{\sigma}\right)\right]^{-1/\xi}\right\}, \quad (3.2)$$

defined on the set $\{z : 1 + \xi(z - \mu)/\sigma > 0\}$, where the parameters satisfy $-\infty < \mu < \infty$, $\sigma > 0$ and $-\infty < \xi < \infty$. This is the **generalized extreme value** (GEV) family of distributions. The model has three parameters: a location parameter, μ; a scale parameter, σ; and a shape parameter, ξ. The type II and type III classes of extreme value distribution correspond respectively to the cases $\xi > 0$ and $\xi < 0$ in this parameterization. The subset of the GEV family with $\xi = 0$ is interpreted as the limit of (3.2) as $\xi \to 0$, leading to the **Gumbel family** with distribution function

$$G(z) = \exp\left[-\exp\left\{-\left(\frac{z-\mu}{\sigma}\right)\right\}\right], \quad -\infty < z < \infty.$$

The unification of the original three families of extreme value distribution into a single family greatly simplifies statistical implementation. Through inference on ξ, the data themselves determine the most appropriate type of tail behavior, and there is no necessity to make subjective a priori judgements about which individual extreme value family to adopt. Moreover, uncertainty in the inferred value of ξ measures the lack of certainty as to which of the original three types is most appropriate for a given dataset.

For convenience we re-state Theorem 3.1 in modified form.

Theorem 3.1.1 If there exist sequences of constants $\{a_n > 0\}$ and $\{b_n\}$ such that

$$\Pr\{(M_n - b_n)/a_n \leq z\} \to G(z) \quad \text{as } n \to \infty \tag{3.3}$$

for a non-degenerate distribution function G, then G is a member of the GEV family

$$G(z) = \exp\left\{-\left[1 + \xi\left(\frac{z-\mu}{\sigma}\right)\right]^{-1/\xi}\right\},$$

defined on $\{z : 1 + \xi(z - \mu)/\sigma > 0\}$, where $-\infty < \mu < \infty$, $\sigma > 0$ and $-\infty < \xi < \infty$. □

Interpreting the limit in Theorem 3.1.1 as an approximation for large values of n suggests the use of the GEV family for modeling the distribution of maxima of long sequences. The apparent difficulty that the normalizing constants will be unknown in practice is easily resolved. Assuming (3.3),

$$\Pr\{(M_n - b_n)/a_n \leq z\} \approx G(z)$$

for large enough n. Equivalently,

$$\Pr\{M_n \leq z\} \approx G\{(z - b_n)/a_n\}$$
$$= G^*(z),$$

where G^* is another member of the GEV family. In other words, if Theorem 3.1.1 enables approximation of the distribution of M_n^* by a member of the

GEV family for large n, the distribution of M_n itself can also be approximated by a different member of the same family. Since the parameters of the distribution have to be estimated anyway, it is irrelevant in practice that the parameters of the distribution G are different from those of G^*.

This argument leads to the following approach for modeling extremes of a series of independent observations $X_1, X_2, \ldots$. Data are blocked into sequences of observations of length n, for some large value of n, generating a series of block maxima, $M_{n,1}, \ldots, M_{n,m}$, say, to which the GEV distribution can be fitted. Often the blocks are chosen to correspond to a time period of length one year, in which case n is the number of observations in a year and the block maxima are annual maxima. Estimates of extreme quantiles of the annual maximum distribution are then obtained by inverting Eq. (3.2):

$$z_p = \begin{cases} \mu - \frac{\sigma}{\xi}\left[1 - \{-\log(1-p)\}^{-\xi}\right], & \text{for } \xi \neq 0, \\ \mu - \sigma \log\{-\log(1-p)\}, & \text{for } \xi = 0, \end{cases} \quad (3.4)$$

where $G(z_p) = 1 - p$. In common terminology, z_p is the **return level** associated with the **return period** $1/p$, since to a reasonable degree of accuracy, the level z_p is expected to be exceeded on average once every $1/p$ years. More precisely, z_p is exceeded by the annual maximum in any particular year with probability p.

Since quantiles enable probability models to be expressed on the scale of data, the relationship of the GEV model to its parameters is most easily interpreted in terms of the quantile expressions (3.4). In particular, defining $y_p = -\log(1-p)$, so that

$$z_p = \begin{cases} \mu - \frac{\sigma}{\xi}\left[1 - y_p^{-\xi}\right], & \text{for } \xi \neq 0, \\ \mu - \sigma \log y_p, & \text{for } \xi = 0, \end{cases}$$

it follows that, if z_p is plotted against y_p on a logarithmic scale – or equivalently, if z_p is plotted against $\log y_p$ – the plot is linear in the case $\xi = 0$. If $\xi < 0$ the plot is convex with asymptotic limit as $p \to 0$ at $\mu - \sigma/\xi$; if $\xi > 0$ the plot is concave and has no finite bound. This graph is a **return level plot**. Because of the simplicity of interpretation, and because the choice of scale compresses the tail of the distribution so that the effect of extrapolation is highlighted, return level plots are particularly convenient for both model presentation and validation. Fig. 3.1 shows return level plots for a range of shape parameters.

3.1.4 Outline Proof of the Extremal Types Theorem

Formal justification of the extremal types theorem is technical, though not especially complicated – see Leadbetter et al. (1983), for example. In this section we give an informal proof. First, it is convenient to make the following definition.

50   3. Classical Extreme Value Theory and Models

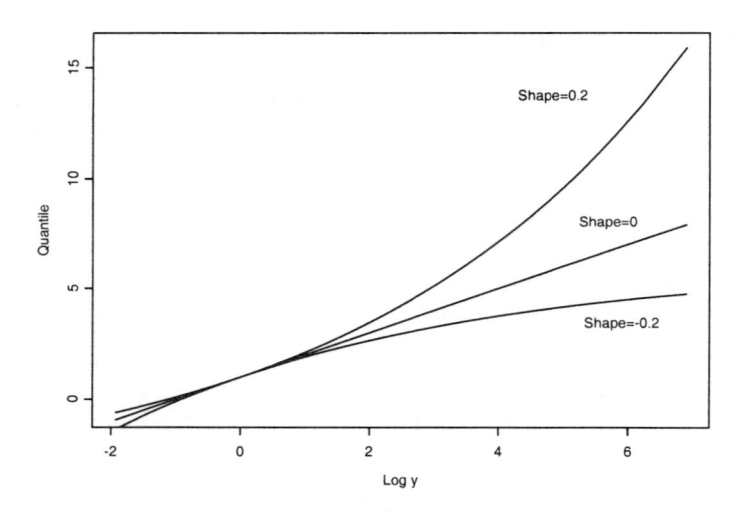

FIGURE 3.1. Return level plots of the GEV distribution with shape parameters $\xi = -0.2$, $\xi = 0$ and $\xi = 0.2$ respectively.

Definition 3.1 A distribution G is said to be **max-stable** if, for every $n = 2, 3, \ldots$, there are constants $\alpha_n > 0$ and β_n such that

$$G^n(\alpha_n z + \beta_n) = G(z).$$

△

Since G^n is the distribution function of $M_n = \max\{X_1, \ldots, X_n\}$, where the X_i are independent variables each having distribution function G, max-stability is a property satisfied by distributions for which the operation of taking sample maxima leads to an identical distribution, apart from a change of scale and location. The connection with the extreme value limit laws is made by the following result.

Theorem 3.2 A distribution is max-stable if, and only if, it is a generalized extreme value distribution.   □

It requires only simple algebra to check that all members of the GEV family are indeed max-stable. The converse requires ideas from functional analysis that are beyond the scope of this book.

Theorem 3.2 is used directly in the proof of the extremal types theorem. The idea is to consider M_{nk}, the maximum random variable in a sequence of $n \times k$ variables for some large value of n. This can be regarded as the maximum of a single sequence of length $n \times k$, or as the maximum of k

maxima, each of which is the maximum of n observations. More precisely, suppose the limit distribution of $(M_n - b_n)/a_n$ is G. So, for large enough n,

$$\Pr\{(M_n - b_n)/a_n \leq z\} \approx G(z)$$

by Theorem 3.1.1. Hence, for any integer k, since nk is large,

$$\Pr\{(M_{nk} - b_{nk})/a_{nk} \leq z\} \approx G(z). \tag{3.5}$$

But, since M_{nk} is the maximum of k variables having the same distribution as M_n,

$$\Pr\{(M_{nk} - b_n)/a_n \leq z\} = [\Pr\{(M_n - b_n)/a_n \leq z\}]^k. \tag{3.6}$$

Hence, by (3.5) and (3.6) respectively,

$$\Pr\{M_{nk} \leq z\} \approx G\left(\frac{z - b_{nk}}{a_{nk}}\right)$$

and

$$\Pr\{M_{nk} \leq z\} \approx G^k\left(\frac{z - b_n}{a_n}\right).$$

Therefore, G and G^k are identical apart from location and scale coefficients. It follows that G is max-stable and therefore a member of the GEV family by Theorem 3.2.

3.1.5 Examples

One issue we have not discussed in connection with Theorem 3.1 is, given a distribution function F, how to establish whether convergence of the distribution of the normalized M_n can actually be achieved. If it can, there are additional questions: what choices of normalizing sequences $\{a_n\}$ and $\{b_n\}$ are necessary and which member of the GEV family is obtained as a limit? Each of the books on extreme value theory referenced in Section 1.4 gives extensive details on these aspects. Since our primary consideration is the statistical inference of real data for which the underlying distribution F is unknown, we will give only a few examples that illustrate how careful choice of normalizing sequences does lead to a limit distribution within the GEV family, as implied by Theorem 3.1. These examples will also be useful for illustrating other limit results in subsequent chapters.

Example 3.1 If $X_1, X_2, \ldots$ is a sequence of independent standard exponential Exp(1) variables, $F(x) = 1 - e^{-x}$ for $x > 0$. In this case, letting

$a_n = 1$ and $b_n = n$,

$$\begin{aligned} \Pr\{(M_n - b_n)/a_n \leq z\} &= F^n(z + \log n) \\ &= \left[1 - e^{-(z+\log n)}\right]^n \\ &= \left[1 - n^{-1}e^{-z}\right]^n \\ &\to \exp(-e^{-z}) \end{aligned}$$

as $n \to \infty$, for each fixed $z \in \mathbb{R}$. Hence, with the chosen a_n and b_n, the limit distribution of M_n as $n \to \infty$ is the Gumbel distribution, corresponding to $\xi = 0$ in the GEV family. ▲

Example 3.2 If $X_1, X_2, \ldots$ is a sequence of independent standard Fréchet variables, $F(x) = \exp(-1/x)$ for $x > 0$. Letting $a_n = n$ and $b_n = 0$,

$$\begin{aligned} \Pr\{(M_n - b_n)/a_n \leq z\} &= F^n(nz) \\ &= [\exp\{-1/(nz)\}]^n \\ &= \exp(-1/z) \end{aligned}$$

as $n \to \infty$, for each fixed $z > 0$. Hence, the limit in this case – which is an exact result for all n, because of the max-stability of F – is also the standard Fréchet distribution: $\xi = 1$ in the GEV family. ▲

Example 3.3 If $X_1, X_2, \ldots$ are a sequence of independent uniform $U(0, 1)$ variables, $F(x) = x$ for $0 \leq x \leq 1$. For fixed $z < 0$, suppose $n > -z$ and let $a_n = 1/n$ and $b_n = 1$. Then,

$$\begin{aligned} \Pr\{(M_n - b_n)/a_n \leq z\} &= F^n(n^{-1}z + 1) \\ &= \left(1 + \frac{z}{n}\right)^n \\ &\to e^z \end{aligned}$$

as $n \to \infty$. Hence, the limit distribution is of Weibull type, with $\xi = -1$ in the GEV family. ▲

There is some latitude in the choice of $\{a_n\}$ and $\{b_n\}$ in such examples. However, different choices that lead to a non-degenerate limit always yield a limit distribution in the GEV family with the same value of ξ, though possibly with other values of the location and scale parameters.

3.2 Asymptotic Models for Minima

Some applications require models for extremely small, rather than extremely large, observations. This is not usually the case for problems involving environmental data, but system failure models, as discussed in Example

1.2, can often be constructed such that the lifetime of a system is equal to the minimum lifetime of a number, n, of individual components. The overall system lifetime is then $\tilde{M}_n = \min\{X_1, \ldots, X_n\}$, where the X_i denote the individual component lifetimes. Assuming the X_i to be independent and identically distributed, analogous arguments apply to $\tilde{M}_n$ as were applied to M_n, leading to a limiting distribution of a suitably re-scaled variable.

The results are also immediate from the corresponding results for M_n. Letting $Y_i = -X_i$ for $i = 1, \ldots, n$, the change of sign means that small values of X_i correspond to large values of Y_i. So if $\tilde{M}_n = \min\{X_1, \ldots, X_n\}$ and $M_n = \max\{Y_1, \ldots, Y_n\}$, then $\tilde{M}_n = -M_n$. Hence, for large n,

$$\begin{aligned}\Pr\{\tilde{M}_n \leq z\} &= \Pr\{-M_n \leq z\} \\ &= \Pr\{M_n \geq -z\} \\ &= 1 - \Pr\{M_n \leq -z\} \\ &\approx 1 - \exp\left\{-\left[1 + \xi\left(\frac{-z-\mu}{\sigma}\right)\right]^{-1/\xi}\right\} \\ &= 1 - \exp\left\{-\left[1 - \xi\left(\frac{z-\tilde{\mu}}{\sigma}\right)\right]^{-1/\xi}\right\},\end{aligned}$$

on $\{z : 1 - \xi(z - \tilde{\mu})/\sigma > 0\}$, where $\tilde{\mu} = -\mu$. This distribution is the **GEV distribution for minima**. We can state the result formally as a theorem analogous to Theorem 3.1.1 for maxima.

Theorem 3.3 *If there exist sequences of constants $\{a_n > 0\}$ and $\{b_n\}$ such that*

$$\Pr\{(\tilde{M}_n - b_n)/a_n \leq z\} \to \tilde{G}(z) \quad \text{as } n \to \infty$$

for a non-degenerate distribution function $\tilde{G}$, then $\tilde{G}$ is a member of the GEV family of distributions for minima:

$$\tilde{G}(z) = 1 - \exp\left\{-\left[1 - \xi\left(\frac{z-\tilde{\mu}}{\sigma}\right)\right]^{-1/\xi}\right\},$$

defined on $\{z : 1 - \xi(z - \tilde{\mu})/\sigma > 0\}$, where $-\infty < \mu < \infty$, $\tilde{\sigma} > 0$ and $-\infty < \xi < \infty$. □

In situations where it is appropriate to model block minima, the GEV distribution for minima can be applied directly. An alternative is to exploit the duality between the distributions for maxima and minima. Given data $z_1, \ldots, z_m$ that are realizations from the GEV distribution for minima, with parameters $(\tilde{\mu}, \sigma, \xi)$, this implies fitting the GEV distribution for maxima to the data $-z_1, \ldots, -z_m$. The maximum likelihood estimate of the parameters of this distribution corresponds exactly to that of the required GEV distribution for minima, apart from the sign correction $\hat{\tilde{\mu}} = -\hat{\mu}$. This approach is used in Section 3.4.2 to model the glass fiber data described in Example 1.2.

3.3 Inference for the GEV Distribution

3.3.1 General Considerations

Motivated by Theorem 3.1.1, the GEV provides a model for the distribution of block maxima. Its application consists of blocking the data into blocks of equal length, and fitting the GEV to the set of block maxima. But in implementing this model for any particular dataset, the choice of block size can be critical. The choice amounts to a trade-off between bias and variance: blocks that are too small mean that approximation by the limit model in Theorem 3.1.1 is likely to be poor, leading to bias in estimation and extrapolation; large blocks generate few block maxima, leading to large estimation variance. Pragmatic considerations often lead to the adoption of blocks of length one year. For example, only the annual maximum data may have been recorded, so that the use of shorter blocks is not an option. Even when this is not the case, an analysis of annual maximum data is likely to be more robust than an analysis based on shorter blocks if the conditions of Theorem 3.1.1 are violated. For example, daily temperatures are likely to vary according to season, violating the assumption that the X_i have a common distribution. If the data were blocked into block lengths of around 3 months, the maximum of the summer block is likely to be much greater than that of the winter block, and an inference that failed to take this non-homogeneity into account would be likely to give inaccurate results. Taking, instead, blocks of length one year means the assumption that individual block maxima have a common distribution is plausible, though the formal justification for the GEV approximation remains invalid.

We now simplify notation by denoting the block maxima $Z_1, \ldots, Z_m$. These are assumed to be independent variables from a GEV distribution whose parameters are to be estimated. If the X_i are independent then the Z_i are also independent. However, independence of the Z_i is likely to be a reasonable approximation even if the X_i constitute a dependent series. In this case, although not covered by Theorem 3.1.1, the conclusion that the Z_i have a GEV distribution may still be reasonable; see Chapter 5.

Many techniques have been proposed for parameter estimation in extreme value models. These include graphical techniques based on versions of probability plots; moment-based techniques in which functions of model moments are equated with their empirical equivalents; procedures in which the parameters are estimated as specified functions of order statistics; and likelihood-based methods. Each technique has its pros and cons, but the all-round utility and adaptability to complex model-building of likelihood-based techniques make this approach particularly attractive.

A potential difficulty with the use of likelihood methods for the GEV concerns the regularity conditions that are required for the usual asymptotic properties associated with the maximum likelihood estimator to be valid. Such conditions are not satisfied by the GEV model because the end-points of the GEV distribution are functions of the parameter values: $\mu - \sigma/\xi$ is an upper end-point of the distribution when $\xi < 0$, and a lower end-point when $\xi > 0$. This violation of the usual regularity conditions means that the standard asymptotic likelihood results are not automatically applicable. Smith (1985) studied this problem in detail and obtained the following results:

- when $\xi > -0.5$, maximum likelihood estimators are regular, in the sense of having the usual asymptotic properties;

- when $-1 < \xi < -0.5$, maximum likelihood estimators are generally obtainable, but do not have the standard asymptotic properties;

- when $\xi < -1$, maximum likelihood estimators are unlikely to be obtainable.

The case $\xi \leq -0.5$ corresponds to distributions with a very short bounded upper tail. This situation is rarely encountered in applications of extreme value modeling, so the theoretical limitations of the maximum likelihood approach are usually no obstacle in practice.

3.3.2 Maximum Likelihood Estimation

Under the assumption that $Z_1, \ldots, Z_m$ are independent variables having the GEV distribution, the log-likelihood for the GEV parameters when $\xi \neq 0$ is

$$\ell(\mu, \sigma, \xi) = -m \log \sigma - (1 + 1/\xi) \sum_{i=1}^{m} \log \left[1 + \xi \left(\frac{z_i - \mu}{\sigma} \right) \right]$$
$$- \sum_{i=1}^{m} \left[1 + \xi \left(\frac{z_i - \mu}{\sigma} \right) \right]^{-1/\xi}, \quad (3.7)$$

provided that

$$1 + \xi \left(\frac{z_i - \mu}{\sigma} \right) > 0, \text{ for } i = 1, \ldots, m. \quad (3.8)$$

At parameter combinations for which (3.8) is violated, corresponding to a configuration for which at least one of the observed data falls beyond an end-point of the distribution, the likelihood is zero and the log-likelihood equals $-\infty$.

The case $\xi = 0$ requires separate treatment using the Gumbel limit of the GEV distribution. This leads to the log-likelihood

$$\ell(\mu, \sigma) = -m \log \sigma - \sum_{i=1}^{m} \left(\frac{z_i - \mu}{\sigma} \right) - \sum_{i=1}^{m} \exp \left\{ -\left(\frac{z_i - \mu}{\sigma} \right) \right\}. \quad (3.9)$$

56   3. Classical Extreme Value Theory and Models

Maximization of the pair of Eqs. (3.7) and (3.9) with respect to the parameter vector (μ, σ, ξ) leads to the maximum likelihood estimate with respect to the entire GEV family. There is no analytical solution, but for any given dataset the maximization is straightforward using standard numerical optimization algorithms. Some care is needed to ensure that such algorithms do not move to parameter combinations violating (3.8), and also that numerical difficulties that would arise from the evaluation of (3.7) in the vicinity of $\xi = 0$ are avoided. This latter problem is easily solved by using (3.9) in place of (3.7) for values of ξ falling within a small window around zero.

Subject to the limitations on ξ discussed in Section 3.3.1, the approximate distribution of $(\hat{\mu}, \hat{\sigma}, \hat{\xi})$ is multivariate normal with mean (μ, σ, ξ) and variance-covariance matrix equal to the inverse of the observed information matrix evaluated at the maximum likelihood estimate. Though this matrix can be calculated analytically, it is easier to use numerical differencing techniques to evaluate the second derivatives, and standard numerical routines to carry out the inversion. Confidence intervals and other forms of inference follow immediately from the approximate normality of the estimator.

3.3.3   Inference for Return Levels

By substitution of the maximum likelihood estimates of the GEV parameters into (3.4), the maximum likelihood estimate of z_p for $0 < p < 1$, the $1/p$ return level, is obtained as

$$\hat{z}_p = \begin{cases} \hat{\mu} - \frac{\hat{\sigma}}{\hat{\xi}}\left[1 - y_p^{-\hat{\xi}}\right], & \text{for } \hat{\xi} \neq 0, \\ \hat{\mu} - \hat{\sigma} \log y_p, & \text{for } \hat{\xi} = 0, \end{cases} \quad (3.10)$$

where $y_p = -\log(1-p)$. Furthermore, by the delta method,

$$\text{Var}(\hat{z}_p) \approx \nabla z_p^T V \nabla z_p, \quad (3.11)$$

where V is the variance-covariance matrix of $(\hat{\mu}, \hat{\sigma}, \hat{\xi})$ and

$$\begin{aligned}\nabla z_p^T &= \left[\frac{\partial z_p}{\partial \mu}, \frac{\partial z_p}{\partial \sigma}, \frac{\partial z_p}{\partial \xi}\right] \\ &= [1, \ -\xi^{-1}(1 - y_p^{-\xi}), \ \sigma\xi^{-2}(1 - y_p^{-\xi}) - \sigma\xi^{-1}y_p^{-\xi}\log y_p]\end{aligned}$$

evaluated at $(\hat{\mu}, \hat{\sigma}, \hat{\xi})$.

It is usually long return periods, corresponding to small values of p, that are of greatest interest. If $\hat{\xi} < 0$ it is also possible to make inferences on the upper end-point of the distribution, which is effectively the 'infinite-observation return period', corresponding to z_p with $p = 0$. The maximum likelihood estimate is

$$\hat{z}_0 = \hat{\mu} - \hat{\sigma}/\hat{\xi},$$

and (3.11) is still valid with

$$\nabla z_0^T = \left[1, \ -\xi^{-1}, \ \sigma\xi^{-2}\right],$$

again evaluated at $(\hat{\mu}, \hat{\sigma}, \hat{\xi})$. When $\hat{\xi} \geq 0$ the maximum likelihood estimate of the upper end-point is infinity.

Caution is required in the interpretation of return level inferences, especially for return levels corresponding to long return periods. First, the normal approximation to the distribution of the maximum likelihood estimator may be poor. Better approximations are generally obtained from the appropriate profile likelihood function; see Section 2.6.6. More fundamentally, estimates and their measures of precision are based on an assumption that the model is correct. Though the GEV model is supported by mathematical argument, its use in extrapolation is based on unverifiable assumptions, and measures of uncertainty on return levels should properly be regarded as lower bounds that could be much greater if uncertainty due to model correctness were taken into account.

3.3.4 Profile Likelihood

Numerical evaluation of the profile likelihood for any of the individual parameters μ, σ or ξ is straightforward. For example, to obtain the profile likelihood for ξ, we fix $\xi = \xi_0$, and maximize the log-likelihood (3.7) with respect to the remaining parameters, μ and σ. This is repeated for a range of values of ξ_0. The corresponding maximized values of the log-likelihood constitute the profile log-likelihood for ξ, from which Theorem 2.6 leads to obtain approximate confidence intervals.

This methodology can also be applied when inference is required on some combination of parameters. In particular, we can obtain confidence intervals for any specified return level z_p. This requires a reparameterization of the GEV model, so that z_p is one of the model parameters, after which the profile log-likelihood is obtained by maximization with respect to the remaining parameters in the usual way. Reparameterization is straightforward:

$$\mu = z_p + \frac{\sigma}{\xi}\left[1 - \{-\log(1-p)\}^{-\xi}\right], \tag{3.12}$$

so that replacement of μ in (3.7) with (3.12) has the desired effect of expressing the GEV model in terms of the parameters (z_p, σ, ξ).

3.3.5 Model Checking

Though it is impossible to check the validity of an extrapolation based on a GEV model, assessment can be made with reference to the observed data. This is not sufficient to justify extrapolation, but is a reasonable prerequisite. In Chapter 2 we discussed the use of probability plots and quantile plots for model checking; we now describe these in more detail for checking the validity of a GEV model, and describe two further graphical goodness-of-fit checks.

As described in Chapter 2, a probability plot is a comparison of the empirical and fitted distribution functions. With ordered block maximum data $z_{(1)} \leq z_{(2)} \leq \cdots \leq z_{(m)}$, the empirical distribution function evaluated at $z_{(i)}$ is given by

$$\tilde{G}(z_{(i)}) = i/(m+1).$$

By substitution of parameter estimates into (3.2), the corresponding model-based estimates are

$$\hat{G}(z_{(i)}) = \exp\left\{-\left[1+\hat{\xi}\left(\frac{z_{(i)}-\hat{\mu}}{\hat{\sigma}}\right)\right]^{-1/\hat{\xi}}\right\}.$$

If the GEV model is working well,

$$\hat{G}(z_{(i)}) \approx \tilde{G}(z_{(i)})$$

for each i, so a probability plot, consisting of the points

$$\left\{\left(\tilde{G}(z_{(i)}), \hat{G}(z_{(i)})\right), i = 1, \ldots, m\right\},$$

should lie close to the unit diagonal. Any substantial departures from linearity are indicative of some failing in the GEV model.

A weakness of the probability plot for extreme value models is that both $\hat{G}(z_{(i)})$ and $\tilde{G}(z_{(i)})$ are bound to approach 1 as $z_{(i)}$ increases, while it is usually the accuracy of the model for large values of z that is of greatest concern. That is, the probability plot provides the least information in the region of most interest. This deficiency is avoided by the quantile plot, consisting of the points

$$\left\{\left(\hat{G}^{-1}(i/(m+1)), z_{(i)}\right), i = 1, \ldots, m\right\}, \qquad (3.13)$$

where, from (3.10),

$$\hat{G}^{-1}\left(\frac{i}{m+1}\right) = \hat{\mu} - \frac{\hat{\sigma}}{\hat{\xi}}\left[1-\left\{-\log\left(\frac{i}{m+1}\right)\right\}^{-\hat{\xi}}\right].$$

Departures from linearity in the quantile plot also indicate model failure.

As discussed in Section 3.1.3, the return level plot, comprising a graph of

$$z_p = \mu - \frac{\sigma}{\xi}\left[1 - \{-\log(1-p)\}^{-\xi}\right]$$

against $y_p = -\log(1-p)$ on a logarithmic scale, is particularly convenient for interpreting extreme value models. The tail of the distribution is compressed, so that return level estimates for long return periods are displayed, while the linearity of the plot in the case $\xi = 0$ provides a baseline against which to judge the effect of the estimated shape parameter.

As a summary of a fitted model the return level plot consists of the locus of points

$$\{(\log y_p, \hat{z}_p) : 0 < p < 1\},$$

where $\hat{z}_p$ is the maximum likelihood estimate of z_p. Confidence intervals can be added to the plot to increase its informativeness. Empirical estimates of the return level function, obtained from the points (3.13), can also be added, enabling the return level plot to be used as a model diagnostic. If the GEV model is suitable for the data, the model-based curve and empirical estimates should be in reasonable agreement. Any substantial or systematic disagreement, after allowance for sampling error, suggests an inadequacy of the GEV model.

The probability, quantile and return level plots are each based on a comparison of model-based and empirical estimates of the distribution function. For completeness, an equivalent diagnostic based on the density function is a comparison of the probability density function of a fitted model with a histogram of the data. This is generally less informative than the previous plots, since the form of a histogram can vary substantially with the choice of grouping intervals. That is, in contrast with the empirical distribution function, there is no unique empirical estimator of a density function, making comparisons with a model-based estimator difficult and subjective.

3.4 Examples

3.4.1 Annual Maximum Sea-levels at Port Pirie

This analysis is based on the series of annual maximum sea-levels recorded at Port Pirie, South Australia, over the period 1923–1987, as described in Example 1.1. From Fig. 1.1 it seems reasonable to assume that the pattern of variation has stayed constant over the observation period, so we model the data as independent observations from the GEV distribution.

Maximization of the GEV log-likelihood for these data leads to the estimate

$$(\hat{\mu}, \hat{\sigma}, \hat{\xi}) = (3.87, 0.198, -0.050),$$

for which the log-likelihood is 4.34. The approximate variance-covariance matrix of the parameter estimates is

$$V = \begin{bmatrix} 0.000780 & 0.000197 & -0.00107 \\ 0.000197 & 0.000410 & -0.000778 \\ -0.00107 & -0.000778 & 0.00965 \end{bmatrix}.$$

The diagonals of the variance-covariance matrix correspond to the variances of the individual parameters of (μ, σ, ξ). Taking square roots, the standard

60   3. Classical Extreme Value Theory and Models

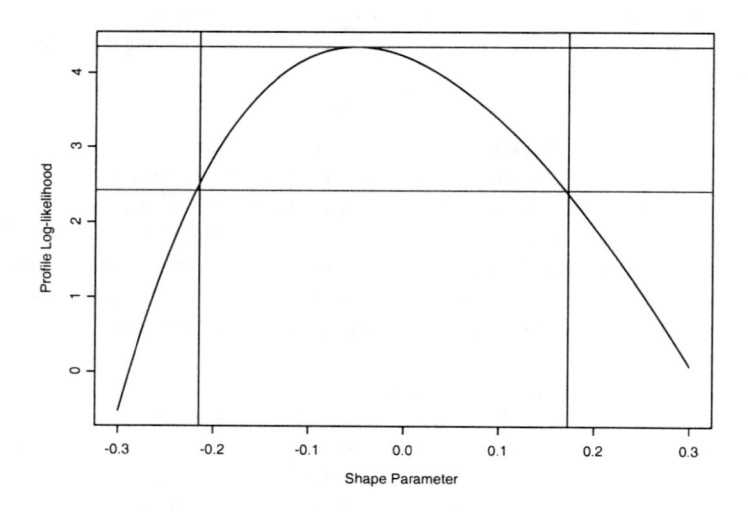

FIGURE 3.2. Profile likelihood for ξ in the Port Pirie sea-level example.

errors are 0.028, 0.020 and 0.098 for $\hat{\mu}, \hat{\sigma}$ and $\hat{\xi}$ respectively. Combining estimates and standard errors, approximate 95% confidence intervals for each parameter are [3.82, 3.93] for μ, [0.158, 0.238] for σ, and [−0.242, 0.142] for ξ. In particular, although the maximum likelihood estimate for ξ is negative, corresponding to a bounded distribution, the 95% confidence interval extends well above zero, so that the strength of evidence from the data for a bounded distribution is not strong. Greater accuracy of confidence intervals can usually be achieved by the use of profile likelihood. Fig. 3.2 shows the profile log-likelihood for ξ, from which a 95% confidence interval for ξ is obtained as [−0.21, 0.17], which is only slightly different to the earlier calculation.

Estimates and confidence intervals for return levels are obtained by substitution into (3.10) and (3.11). For example, to estimate the 10-year return level, we set $p = 1/10$ and find $\hat{z}_{0.1} = 4.30$ and $\text{Var}(\hat{z}_{0.1}) = 0.00303$. Hence, a 95% confidence interval for $z_{0.1}$ is evaluated as $4.30 \pm 1.96 \times \sqrt{0.00303} =$ [4.19, 4.41]. The corresponding estimate for the 100-year return level is $\hat{z}_{0.01} = 4.69$, with a 95% confidence interval of [4.38, 5.00].

Better accuracy again comes from the profile likelihood. Figs. 3.3 and 3.4 show the profile log-likelihood for the 10- and 100-year return levels respectively. By Theorem 2.6 we obtain confidence intervals for $z_{0.1}$ and $z_{0.01}$ of [4.21, 4.45] and [4.50, 5.27] respectively. The first of these is similar to that obtained from the delta method, while the second is not. The latter discrepancy arises because of asymmetry in the profile log-likelihood surface, the extent of which increases with increasing return period. Such

3.4 Examples 61

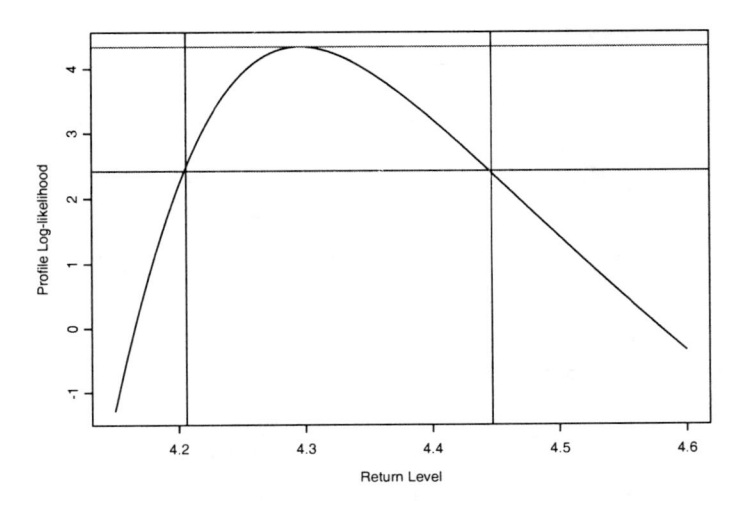

FIGURE 3.3. Profile likelihood for 10-year return level in the Port Pirie sea-level example.

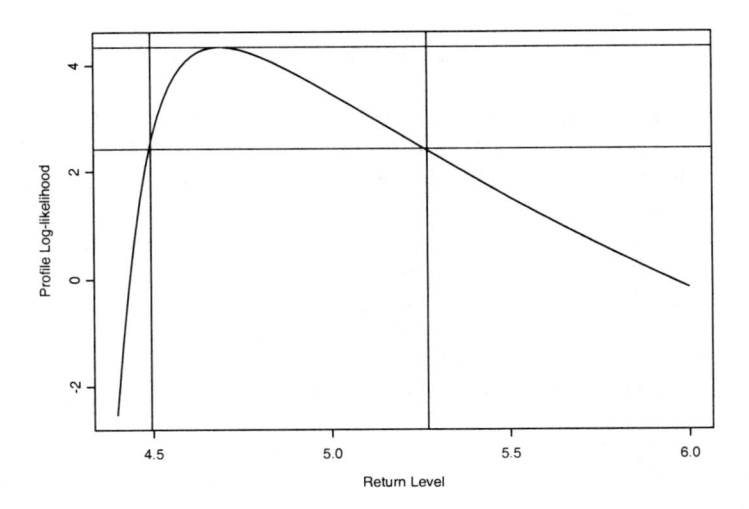

FIGURE 3.4. Profile likelihood for 100-year return level in the Port Pirie sea-level example.

62   3. Classical Extreme Value Theory and Models

asymmetries are to be expected, since the data provide increasingly weaker information about high levels of the process.

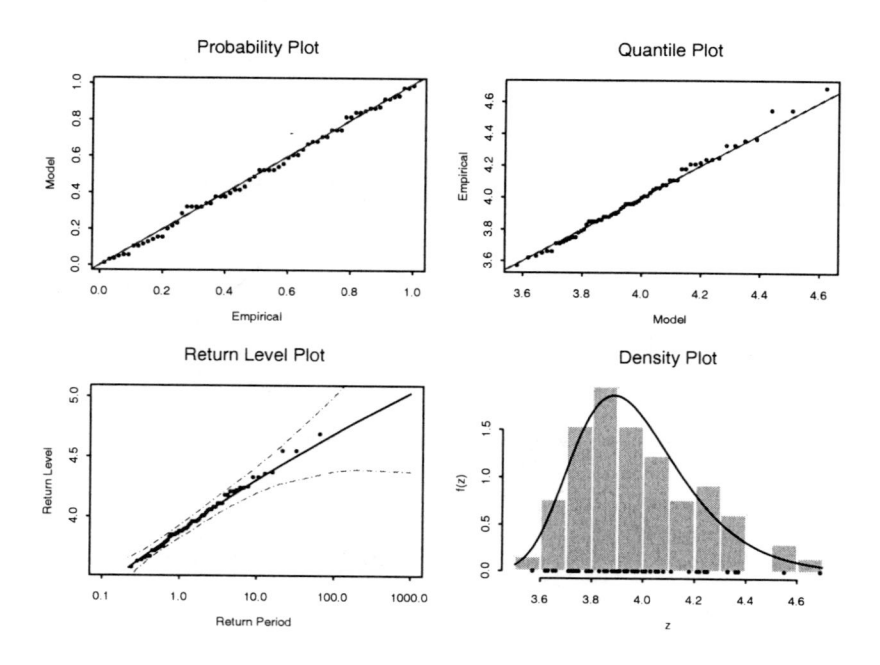

FIGURE 3.5. Diagnostic plots for GEV fit to the Port Pirie sea-level data.

The various diagnostic plots for assessing the accuracy of the GEV model fitted to the Port Pirie data are shown in Fig. 3.5. Neither the probability plot nor the quantile plot give cause to doubt the validity of the fitted model: each set of plotted points is near-linear. The return level curve asymptotes to a finite level as a consequence of the negative estimate of ξ, though since the estimate is close to zero, the estimated curve is close to linear. The curve also provides a satisfactory representation of the empirical estimates, especially once sampling variability is taken into account. Finally, the corresponding density estimate seems consistent with the histogram of the data. Consequently, all four diagnostic plots lend support to the fitted GEV model.

The original version of the extremal types theorem, as given in Theorem 3.1, identifies three possible families of limit distributions for maxima. Before the unification of the three distributions into the single GEV family, it was natural to make a preliminary choice of model type prior to parameter estimation. This approach now has little merit, given the alternative option of modeling within the entire GEV family. However, the suitability of any particular member of the GEV family can be assessed by comparison with the maximum likelihood estimate within the entire family. For example, the appropriateness of replacing the GEV family with the Gumbel family, corresponding to the $\xi = 0$ subset of the GEV family, can be assessed.

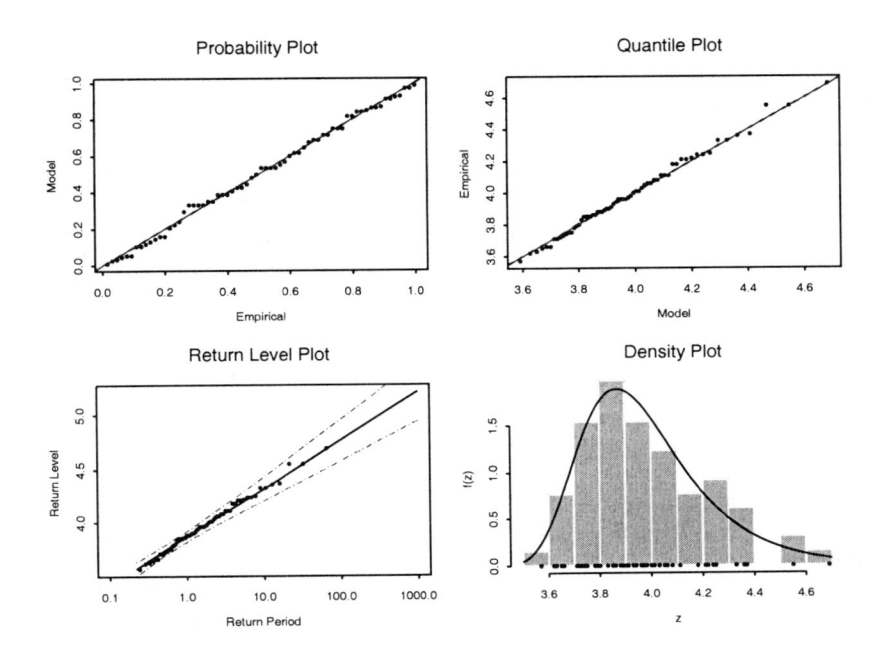

FIGURE 3.6. Diagnostic plots for Gumbel fit to the Port Pirie sea-level data.

Maximum likelihood in the Gumbel case corresponds to maximization of (3.9), followed by standard treatment to obtain standard errors etc. For the Port Pirie sea-level data this leads to $(\hat{\mu}, \hat{\sigma}) = (3.87, 0.195)$, with standard errors 0.03 and 0.019 respectively. The maximized log-likelihood is -4.22. The likelihood ratio test statistic for the reduction to the Gumbel model is therefore $D = 2\{-4.22 - (-4.34)\} = 0.24$. This value is small when compared to the χ_1^2 distribution, suggesting that the Gumbel model is adequate for these data. This is confirmed by the standard diagnostic graphical checks in Fig. 3.6, which imply that the goodness-of-fit is comparable with that of the GEV model. This is not surprising since the estimated parameters in the two models are so similar, which also means that (short-term) model extrapolation on the basis of either model leads to similar answers. The greatest difference between the two models is in terms of the precision of estimation: the model parameters and return levels have estimates with considerably shorter confidence intervals in the Gumbel model, compared with the GEV model.

The issue of choice between the Gumbel and GEV models is starkly illustrated by the respective return level plots of Figs. 3.5 and 3.6. The estimated return level curves are similar, but the confidence intervals are much wider for the GEV model, especially for long return periods. Reduction of uncertainty is desirable, so that if the Gumbel model could be trusted, its inferences would be preferred. But can the model be trusted? The extremal types theorem provides support for modeling block maxima with the GEV family, of which the Gumbel family is a subset. The data suggest that a Gumbel model is plausible, but this does not imply that other models are not. Indeed, the maximum likelihood estimate within the GEV family is not in the Gumbel family (although, in the sense that $\hat{\xi} \approx 0$, it is 'close'). There is no common agreement about this issue, but the safest option is to accept there is uncertainty about the value of the shape parameter – and hence whether the Gumbel model is correct or not – and to prefer the inference based on the GEV model. The larger measures of uncertainty generated by the GEV model then provide more a realistic quantification of the genuine uncertainties involved in model extrapolation.

3.4.2 Glass Fiber Strength Example

We now consider the glass fiber breaking strength data of Example 1.2. For the reasons discussed in Section 3.2, the GEV model for minima is an appropriate starting point for data of this type. There are two equivalent approaches to the modeling. Either the GEV distribution for minima can be fitted directly to the data, or the data can be negated and the GEV distribution for maxima fitted to these data. The equivalence of these operations is justified in Section 3.2. To economize on the writing of model-fitting routines, we take the approach of fitting the GEV distribution to the negated data. This leads to the maximum likelihood estimate

$$(\hat{\mu}, \hat{\sigma}, \hat{\xi}) = (-1.64, 0.27, -0.084),$$

with a maximized value of the log-likelihood equal to -14.3. The corresponding estimated variance-covariance matrix is

$$V = \begin{bmatrix} 0.00141 & 0.000214 & -0.000795 \\ 0.000214 & 0.000652 & -0.000441 \\ -0.000795 & -0.0000441 & 0.00489 \end{bmatrix}.$$

Taking square roots of the diagonals of this matrix leads to standard errors of μ, σ and ξ as $0.038, 0.026$ and 0.070 respectively. The estimates and standard errors combine to give approximate confidence intervals. In particular, a 95% confidence interval for ξ is obtained as $-0.084 \pm 1.96 \times 0.07 = [-0.22, 0.053]$. So, as in the previous example, the maximum likelihood estimate of the shape parameter is negative, but both negative and positive values are plausible once sampling uncertainty is accounted for.

3.4 Examples 65

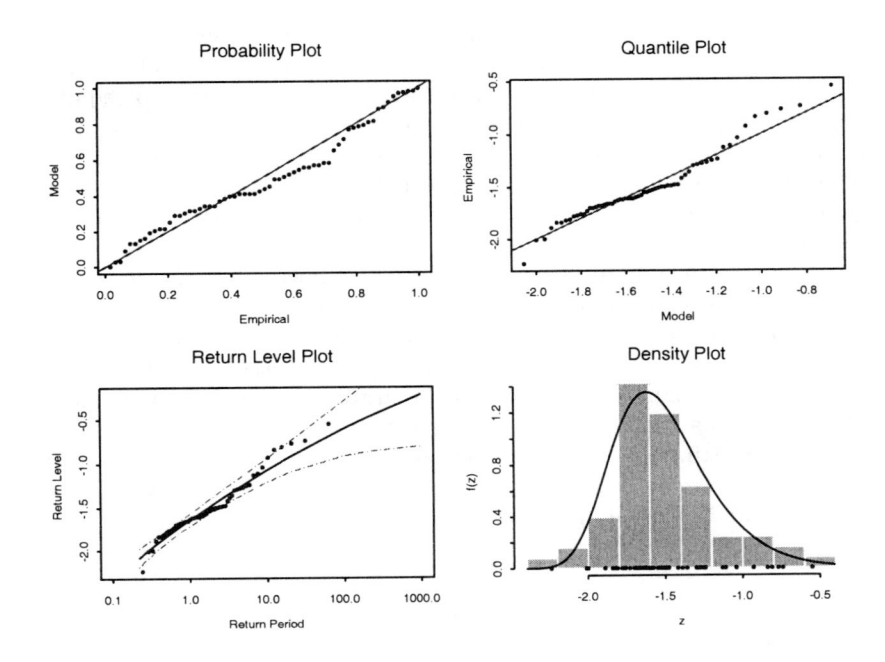

FIGURE 3.7. Diagnostic plots of GEV fit to negative breaking strengths of glass fibers.

From Section 3.2 the estimates for the parameters $(\tilde{\mu}, \sigma, \xi)$ of the corresponding GEV distribution for minima applied directly to the original data are

$$(\hat{\tilde{\mu}}, \hat{\sigma}, \hat{\xi}) = (1.64, 0.27, -0.084).$$

The change of sign of the location parameter induces a change to the sign of appropriate components of the variance-covariance matrix, which now becomes

$$V = \begin{bmatrix} 0.00141 & -0.000214 & 0.000795 \\ -0.000214 & 0.000652 & -0.000441 \\ 0.000795 & -0.0000441 & 0.00489 \end{bmatrix}.$$

Returning to the GEV analysis, the diagnostic plots for the fitted model are shown in Fig. 3.7. The probability and quantile plots are less convincing than in the previous example, but there is less doubt about the quality of fit once confidence intervals are added to the return level curve.

Interpretation of return levels in this example needs some explanation. The "return period" of 1000 has a "return level" of around -0.4. Such terminology doesn't work so well here; the values imply that, given 1000 such glass fibers, just one would be expected to have a breaking strength below

0.4 units. This point also raises an issue that is often used as an objection to the use of the GEV family. Looking at the return level plot in Fig. 3.7, it is clear that the model extrapolates to positive values, or equivalently, to negative values of breaking strength. This is incompatible with the physical process under study. In fact, the estimated upper end-point of the fitted distribution is $\hat{z}_0 = \hat{\mu} - \hat{\sigma}/\hat{\xi} = 1.59$, corresponding to a breaking strength of -1.59 units. The situation would be worse had the estimate of ξ been non-negative, since the estimated upper end-point of the distribution would have been infinite. This situation is not uncommon. For example, GEV estimates of annual maxima of daily rainfall often lead to positive estimates of ξ, though it is unreasonable on physical grounds to believe that daily rainfall levels are truly without limit. What these arguments really illustrate is the danger of relying on the arguments leading to the GEV distribution as a basis for very long-term extrapolation. Although the arguments for fitting the GEV distribution to block maxima are compelling, the temptation to extrapolate to extremely high levels should be tempered by caution and physical knowledge.

3.5 Model Generalization: the r Largest Order Statistic Model

3.5.1 Model Formulation

An implicit difficulty in any extreme value analysis is the limited amount of data for model estimation. Extremes are scarce, by definition, so that model estimates, especially of extreme return levels, have a large variance. This issue has motivated the search for characterizations of extreme value behavior that enable the modeling of data other than just block maxima.

There are two well-known general characterizations. One is based on exceedances of a high threshold, the other is based on the behavior of the r largest order statistics within a block, for small values of r. Both characterizations can be unified using a point process representation discussed in Chapter 7. In this section we focus on a model for the r largest order statistics.

As in previous sections, we suppose that $X_1, X_2, \ldots$ is a sequence of independent and identically distributed random variables, and aim to characterize the extremal behavior of the X_i. In Section 3.1.3 we obtained that the limiting distribution as $n \to \infty$ of M_n, suitably re-scaled, is GEV. We first extend this result to other extreme order statistics, by defining

$$M_n^{(k)} = k\text{th largest of } \{X_1, \ldots, X_n\},$$

and identifying the limiting behavior of this variable, for fixed k, as $n \to \infty$. The following result generalizes Theorem 3.1.

3.5 Model Generalization: the r Largest Order Statistic Model

Theorem 3.4 If there exist sequences of constants $\{a_n > 0\}$ and $\{b_n\}$ such that
$$\Pr\{(M_n - b_n)/a_n \leq z\} \to G(z) \quad \text{as } n \to \infty$$
for some non-degenerate distribution function G, so that G is the GEV distribution function given by (3.2), then, for fixed k,
$$\Pr\{(M_n^{(k)} - b_n)/a_n \leq z\} \to G_k(z)$$
on $\{z : 1 + \xi(z - \mu)/\sigma > 0\}$, where
$$G_k(z) = \exp\{-\tau(z)\} \sum_{s=0}^{k-1} \frac{\tau(z)^s}{s!} \tag{3.14}$$
with
$$\tau(z) = \left[1 + \xi \left(\frac{z - \mu}{\sigma}\right)\right]^{-1/\xi}.$$

□

Theorem 3.4 implies that, if the kth largest order statistic in a block is normalized in exactly the same way as the maximum, then its limiting distribution is of the form given by (3.14), the parameters of which correspond to the parameters of the limiting GEV distribution of the block maximum. Again, by absorbing the unknown scaling constants into the model location and scale parameters, it follows that, for large n, the approximate distribution of $M_n^{(k)}$ is within the family (3.14).

There is, however, a difficulty in using (3.14) as a model. The situation we are often faced with, as with the Venice sea-level example, is of having each of the largest r order statistics within each of several blocks, for some value of r. That is, we usually have the complete vector
$$\boldsymbol{M}_n^{(r)} = (M_n^{(1)}, \ldots, M_n^{(r)})$$
for each of several blocks. In the case of the Venice sea-level data, $r = 10$ for most of the blocks, each of which corresponds to one year of observations. Whilst Theorem 3.4 gives a family for the approximate distribution of each of the components of $\boldsymbol{M}_n^{(r)}$, it does not give the joint distribution of $\boldsymbol{M}_n^{(r)}$. Moreover, the components cannot be independent: $M_n^{(2)}$ can be no greater than $M_n^{(1)}$, for example, so the outcome of each component influences the distribution of the other. Consequently, the result of Theorem 3.4 does not in itself lead to a model for $\boldsymbol{M}_n^{(r)}$. Instead, we require a characterization of the limiting joint distribution of the entire vector $\boldsymbol{M}_n^{(r)}$. With appropriate re-scaling this can be achieved, but the limiting joint distribution it leads to is intractable. However, the following theorem gives the joint density function of the limit distribution.

68   3. Classical Extreme Value Theory and Models

Theorem 3.5 If there exist sequences of constants $\{a_n > 0\}$ and $\{b_n\}$ such that
$$\Pr\{(M_n - b_n)/a_n \leq z\} \to G(z) \quad \text{as } n \to \infty$$
for some non-degenerate distribution function G, then, for fixed r, the limiting distribution as $n \to \infty$ of
$$\tilde{M}_n^{(r)} = \left(\frac{M_n^{(1)} - b_n}{a_n}, \ldots, \frac{M_n^{(r)} - b_n}{a_n}\right)$$
falls within the family having joint probability density function
$$f(z^{(1)}, \ldots, z^{(r)}) = \exp\left\{-\left[1 + \xi\left(\frac{z^{(r)} - \mu}{\sigma}\right)\right]^{-1/\xi}\right\}$$
$$\times \prod_{k=1}^{r} \sigma^{-1}\left[1 + \xi\left(\frac{z^{(k)} - \mu}{\sigma}\right)\right]^{-\frac{1}{\xi} - 1}, \quad (3.15)$$
where $-\infty < \mu < \infty$, $\sigma > 0$ and $-\infty < \xi < \infty$; $z^{(r)} \leq z^{(r-1)} \leq \cdots \leq z^{(1)}$; and $z^{(k)} : 1 + \xi(z^{(k)} - \mu)/\sigma > 0$ for $k = 1, \ldots, r$. □

Proofs of Theorems 3.4 and 3.5 are given in Chapter 7. In the case $r = 1$, (3.15) reduces to the GEV family of density functions. The case $\xi = 0$ in (3.15) is interpreted as the limiting form as $\xi \to 0$, leading to the family of density functions
$$f(z^{(1)}, \ldots, z^{(r)}) = \exp\left\{-\exp\left[-\left(\frac{z^{(r)} - \mu}{\sigma}\right)\right]\right\}$$
$$\times \prod_{k=1}^{r} \sigma^{-1} \exp\left[-\left(\frac{z^{(k)} - \mu}{\sigma}\right)\right], \quad (3.16)$$
for which the case $r = 1$ reduces to the density of the Gumbel family.

3.5.2 Modeling the r Largest Order Statistics

Starting with a series of independent and identically distributed variables, data are grouped into m blocks. In block i the largest r_i observations are recorded, leading to the series $M_i^{(r_i)} = (z_i^{(1)}, \ldots, z_i^{(r_i)})$, for $i = 1, \ldots, m$. It is usual to set $r_1 = \cdots = r_m = r$ for some specified value of r, unless fewer data are available in some blocks.

As with the GEV model, the issue of block size amounts to a trade-off between bias and variance that is usually resolved by making a pragmatic choice, such as a block size of length one year. The number of order statistics used in each block also comprises a bias-variance trade-off: small values of

3.5 Model Generalization: the r Largest Order Statistic Model

r generate few data leading to high variance; large values of r are likely to violate the asymptotic support for the model, leading to bias. In practice it is usual to select the r_i as large as possible, subject to adequate model diagnostics.

The likelihood for this model is obtained from (3.15) and (3.16), by absorbing the unknown scaling coefficients into location and scale parameters in the usual way, and by taking products across blocks. So, when $\xi \neq 0$,

$$L(\mu, \sigma, \xi) = \prod_{i=1}^{m} \left(\exp\left\{ -\left[1 + \xi \left(\frac{z_i^{(r_i)} - \mu}{\sigma}\right)\right]^{-1/\xi} \right\} \right.$$
$$\left. \times \prod_{k=1}^{r_i} \sigma^{-1} \left[1 + \xi \left(\frac{z_i^{(k)} - \mu}{\sigma}\right)\right]^{-\frac{1}{\xi} - 1} \right), \quad (3.17)$$

provided $1 + \xi(z^{(k)} - \mu)/\sigma > 0$, $k = 1, \ldots, r_i, i = 1, \ldots, m$; otherwise the likelihood is zero. When $\xi = 0$,

$$L(\mu, \sigma, \xi) = \prod_{i=1}^{m} \left(\exp\left\{ -\exp\left[-\left(\frac{z_i^{(r_i)} - \mu}{\sigma}\right)\right]\right\} \right.$$
$$\left. \times \prod_{k=1}^{r_i} \sigma^{-1} \exp\left[-\left(\frac{z_i^{(k)} - \mu}{\sigma}\right)\right] \right). \quad (3.18)$$

The likelihood (3.17) and (3.18) or, more commonly, the corresponding log-likelihood, can be maximized numerically to obtain maximum likelihood estimates. Standard asymptotic likelihood theory also gives approximate standard errors and confidence intervals. In the special case of $r_i = 1$ for each i, the likelihood function reduces to the likelihood of the GEV model for block maxima. More generally, the r largest order statistic model gives a likelihood whose parameters correspond to those of the GEV distribution of block maxima, but which incorporates more of the observed extreme data. So, relative to a standard block maxima analysis, the interpretation of the parameters is unaltered, but precision should be improved due to the inclusion of extra information.

3.5.3 Venice Sea-level Data

These data, discussed in Example 1.5, consist of the 10 largest sea-levels in Venice over the period 1931–1981, except for the year 1935, for which only the largest 6 observations are available. So, with due allowance for the exceptional year, model (3.15) can be applied for any value of $r = 1, \ldots, 10$. Maximum likelihood estimates and standard errors are given in Table 3.1 for inferences based on selected values of r. As anticipated, with increasing

70   3. Classical Extreme Value Theory and Models

TABLE 3.1. Maximized log-likelihoods ℓ, parameter estimates and standard errors (in parentheses) of r largest order statistic model fitted to the Venice sea-level data with different values of r.

r	ℓ	$\hat{\mu}$	$\hat{\sigma}$	$\hat{\xi}$
1	−222.7	111.1 (2.6)	17.2 (1.8)	−0.077 (0.074)
5	−732.0	118.6 (1.6)	13.7 (0.8)	−0.088 (0.033)
10	−1149.3	120.4 (1.3)	12.7 (0.5)	−0.115 (0.019)

values of r, the standard errors decrease, corresponding to increased model precision. However, if the asymptotic approximation is valid for a particular choice of r, then parameter estimates should be stable when the model is fitted with fewer order statistics. But from Table 3.1, there is little evidence of stability in the location and scale parameter estimates, even once sampling variability is accounted for. This brings into doubt the validity of the model, at least for values of $r \geq 5$.

Since the parameters μ, σ and ξ correspond exactly to the GEV parameters of the annual maxima distribution, a more detailed assessment of model fit is derived from return level curves of the annual maximum distribution. These are constructed in exactly the same way as for the block maximum model, but this time using the maximum likelihood estimates and variance-covariance matrix from the r largest order statistic model. Fig. 3.8 shows these plots for each value of r from 2 to 10. Even in the case of $r = 2$, the fit is not particularly good; the reasons for this will be discussed in Chapter 6. Notwithstanding general concerns about the lack of fit, Fig. 3.8 also illustrates that the agreement between model and data diminishes as r increases, although the confidence intervals become less wide. This is a graphic illustration of the bias-variance trade-off determined by the choice of r.

For any particular choice of r, the accuracy of the fit can also be examined in greater detail. First, the complete range of diagnostics for the block maximum can be examined. As an example, with $r = 5$, the usual suite of annual maximum diagnostics is shown in Fig. 3.9. Like the return level plots, these are obtained in exactly the same way as for the block maximum model, substituting the parameter estimates and variance-covariance matrix with those obtained by the maximization of (3.17). For the Venice data, the concern for lack of fit is reinforced by these diagnostics. Checks can also be made on the quality of fit for each of the order statistics by plotting probability and quantile plots. These are obtained by comparing the distribution of the kth order statistic – model (3.14), with parameter values replaced by their estimates – with the corresponding empirical estimates. For the probability plot this is straightforward. The quantile plot is more complicated, since (3.14) cannot be analytically inverted and it is

3.5 Model Generalization: the r Largest Order Statistic Model 71

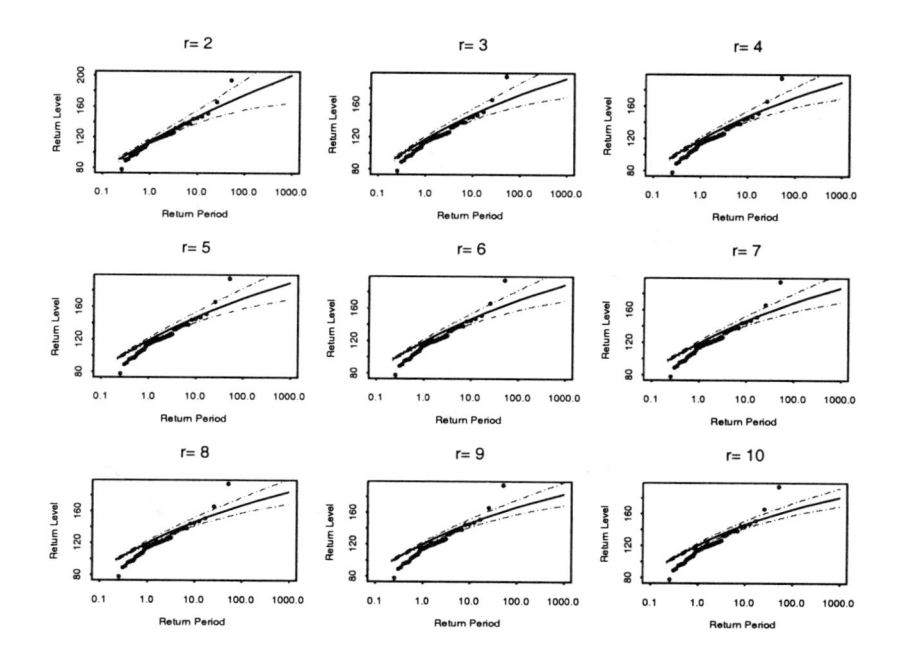

FIGURE 3.8. Return level estimates with 95% confidence intervals for annual maxima distribution based on r largest order statistic model fitted to the Venice sea-level data.

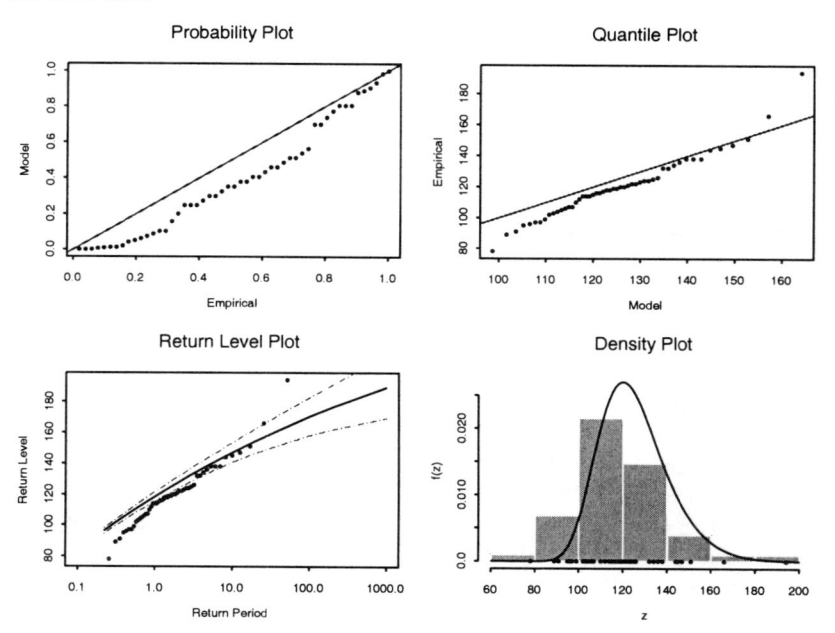

FIGURE 3.9. Annual maximum GEV diagnostics for the Venice sea-level data on basis of fitted r largest order statistic model with $r = 5$.

72   3. Classical Extreme Value Theory and Models

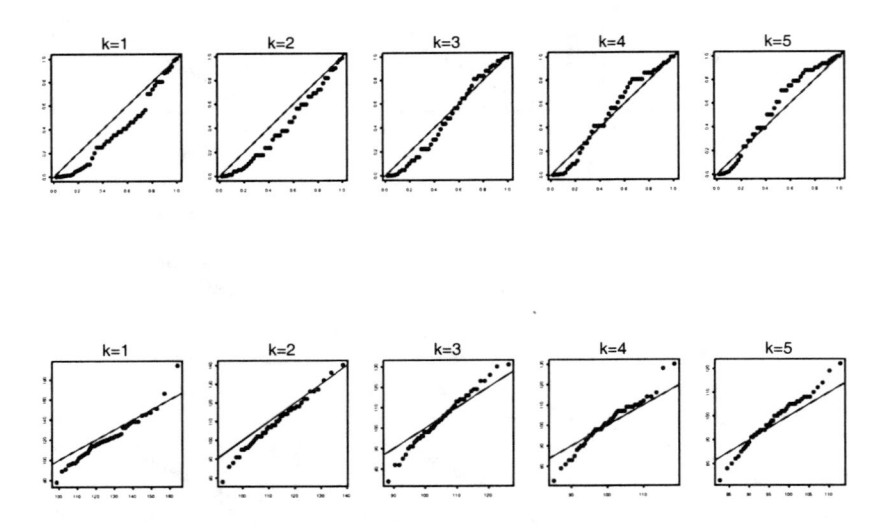

FIGURE 3.10. Model diagnostics for the Venice sea-level data on basis of fitted r largest order statistic model with $r = 5$. Plots shown are probability plots (top row) and quantile plots (bottom row) for kth largest order statistic, $k = 1, \ldots, 5$.

necessary to solve numerically the equation

$$G_k(z_p) = 1 - p$$

to obtain the model estimate of the $1 - p$ quantile. Nonetheless, this is straightforward using standard numerical techniques. For the Venice data, with the fitted model corresponding to $r = 5$, probability and quantile plots for each of the four largest order statistics are given in Fig. 3.10. These plots again indicate a fundamental lack of fit for the model.

3.6 Further Reading

The origins of the asymptotic sample maximum characterization can be traced back to Fisher & Tippett (1928). Their arguments were completed and formalized by Gnedenko (1943). Serious use of the block maximum model for statistical applications seems only to have started in the 1950's. Gumbel (1958) was influential in promoting the methodology, and this book is still relevant today. The GEV parameterization of the extreme value limit models was independently proposed by von Mises (1954) and Jenkinson (1955).

Aspects of likelihood inference for the GEV model, and in particular the calculation of the expected information matrix, were considered by Prescott & Walden (1980); this was subsequently generalized to the case of censored data by Prescott & Walden (1983). An explicit algorithm for estimating maximum likelihood parameters was given by Hosking (1985). Smith (1985) contains important calculations for establishing the asymptotic properties of the maximum likelihood estimator for a class of models that includes the GEV. The issue of testing for the Gumbel model as a special case of the GEV distribution is discussed by Hosking (1984).

Competitor methods to maximum likelihood for estimating the parameters of the GEV distribution include the technique of probability weighted moments (Hosking et al., 1985) and methods based on order statistics (de Haan, 1990). Modified moment and likelihood techniques have also been proposed in a series of articles by JP Cohen: see Cohen (1988) for an overview and Smith (1995) for a general discussion and comparison.

There are numerous published applications of the GEV model in a variety of disciplines. A number of recent publications were listed in Section 1.1. Other influential examples include Buishand (1989) and Carter & Challenor (1981) for climatology; de Haan (1990), Tawn (1992) and Robinson & Tawn (1997) for oceanography; Zwiers (1987) and Walshaw & Anderson (2000) for wind field modeling; Henery (1984) and Robinson & Tawn (1995) for sports data modeling. The connections between extreme value models and reliability models are discussed in detail by Crowder et al. (1991). Applications in the context of corrosion engineering are described by Scarf & Laycock (1996).

Examples based on the r largest order statistic model are less common. As a modeling tool, the technique was first developed in the Gumbel case of $\xi = 0$ by Smith (1986), building on theoretical developments in Weissman (1978). The general case, having arbitrary ξ, was developed by Tawn (1988b).

4
Threshold Models

4.1 Introduction

As discussed in Chapter 3, modeling only block maxima is a wasteful approach to extreme value analysis if other data on extremes are available. Though the r largest order statistic model is a better alternative, it is unusual to have data of this form. Moreover, even this method can be wasteful of data if one block happens to contain more extreme events than another. If an entire time series of, say, hourly or daily observations is available, then better use is made of the data by avoiding altogether the procedure of blocking.

Let $X_1, X_2, \ldots$ be a sequence of independent and identically distributed random variables, having marginal distribution function F. It is natural to regard as extreme events those of the X_i that exceed some high threshold u. Denoting an arbitrary term in the X_i sequence by X, it follows that a description of the stochastic behavior of extreme events is given by the conditional probability

$$\Pr\{X > u + y \mid X > u\} = \frac{1 - F(u+y)}{1 - F(u)}, \quad y > 0. \tag{4.1}$$

If the parent distribution F were known, the distribution of threshold exceedances in (4.1) would also be known. Since, in practical applications, this is not the case, approximations that are broadly applicable for high values of the threshold are sought. This parallels the use of the GEV as an approximation to the distribution of maxima of long sequences when the parent population is unknown.

4.2 Asymptotic Model Characterization

4.2.1 The Generalized Pareto Distribution

The main result is contained in the following theorem.

Theorem 4.1 Let $X_1, X_2, \ldots$ be a sequence of independent random variables with common distribution function F, and let

$$M_n = \max\{X_1, \ldots, X_n\}.$$

Denote an arbitrary term in the X_i sequence by X, and suppose that F satisfies Theorem 3.1.1, so that for large n,

$$\Pr\{M_n \leq z\} \approx G(z),$$

where

$$G(z) = \exp\left\{-\left[1 + \xi\left(\frac{z-\mu}{\sigma}\right)\right]^{-1/\xi}\right\}$$

for some $\mu, \sigma > 0$ and ξ. Then, for large enough u, the distribution function of $(X - u)$, conditional on $X > u$, is approximately

$$H(y) = 1 - \left(1 + \frac{\xi y}{\tilde{\sigma}}\right)^{-1/\xi} \tag{4.2}$$

defined on $\{y : y > 0 \text{ and } (1 + \xi y/\tilde{\sigma}) > 0\}$, where

$$\tilde{\sigma} = \sigma + \xi(u - \mu). \tag{4.3}$$

□

Theorem 4.1 can also be made more precise, justifying (4.2) as a limiting distribution as u increases. In Section 4.2.2 we give an outline proof of the theorem as stated here.

The family of distributions defined by Eq. (4.2) is called the **generalized Pareto family**. Theorem 4.1 implies that, if block maxima have approximating distribution G, then threshold excesses have a corresponding approximate distribution within the generalized Pareto family. Moreover, the parameters of the generalized Pareto distribution of threshold excesses are uniquely determined by those of the associated GEV distribution of block maxima. In particular, the parameter ξ in (4.2) is equal to that of the corresponding GEV distribution. Choosing a different, but still large, block size n would affect the values of the GEV parameters, but not those of the corresponding generalized Pareto distribution of threshold excesses: ξ is invariant to block size, while the calculation of $\tilde{\sigma}$ in (4.3) is unperturbed by the changes in μ and σ which are self-compensating.

The duality between the GEV and generalized Pareto families means that the shape parameter ξ is dominant in determining the qualitative behavior of the generalized Pareto distribution, just as it is for the GEV distribution. If $\xi < 0$ the distribution of excesses has an upper bound of $u - \tilde{\sigma}/\xi$; if $\xi > 0$ the distribution has no upper limit. The distribution is also unbounded if $\xi = 0$, which should again be interpreted by taking the limit $\xi \to 0$ in (4.2), leading to

$$H(y) = 1 - \exp\left(-\frac{y}{\tilde{\sigma}}\right), \quad y > 0, \tag{4.4}$$

corresponding to an exponential distribution with parameter $1/\tilde{\sigma}$.

4.2.2 Outline Justification for the Generalized Pareto Model

This section provides an outline proof of Theorem 4.1. A more precise argument is given by Leadbetter et al. (1983).

Let X have distribution function F. By the assumption of Theorem 3.1, for large enough n,

$$F^n(z) \approx \exp\left\{-\left[1 + \xi\left(\frac{z-\mu}{\sigma}\right)\right]^{-1/\xi}\right\}$$

for some parameters $\mu, \sigma > 0$ and ξ. Hence,

$$n \log F(z) \approx -\left[1 + \xi\left(\frac{z-\mu}{\sigma}\right)\right]^{-1/\xi}. \tag{4.5}$$

But for large values of z, a Taylor expansion implies that

$$\log F(z) \approx -\{1 - F(z)\}.$$

Substitution into (4.5), followed by rearrangement, gives

$$1 - F(u) \approx \frac{1}{n}\left[1 + \xi\left(\frac{u-\mu}{\sigma}\right)\right]^{-1/\xi}$$

for large u. Similarly, for $y > 0$,

$$1 - F(u+y) \approx \frac{1}{n}\left[1 + \xi\left(\frac{u+y-\mu}{\sigma}\right)\right]^{-1/\xi}. \tag{4.6}$$

Hence,

$$\Pr\{X > u + y \mid X > u\} \approx \frac{n^{-1}\left[1 + \xi(u + y - \mu)/\sigma\right]^{-1/\xi}}{n^{-1}\left[1 + \xi(u - \mu)/\sigma\right]^{-1/\xi}}$$

$$= \left[1 + \frac{\xi(u + y - \mu)/\sigma}{1 + \xi(u - \mu)/\sigma}\right]^{-1/\xi}$$

$$= \left[1 + \frac{\xi y}{\tilde{\sigma}}\right]^{-1/\xi}, \qquad (4.7)$$

where

$$\tilde{\sigma} = \sigma + \xi(u - \mu),$$

as required.

4.2.3 Examples

We now reconsider the three theoretical examples of Section 3.1.5 in terms of threshold exceedance models.

Example 4.1 For the exponential model, $F(x) = 1 - e^{-x}$, for $x > 0$. By direct calculation,

$$\frac{1 - F(u + y)}{1 - F(u)} = \frac{e^{-(u+y)}}{e^{-u}} = e^{-y}$$

for all $y > 0$. Consequently, the limit distribution of threshold exceedances is the exponential distribution, corresponding to $\xi = 0$ and $\tilde{\sigma} = 1$ in the generalized Pareto family. Furthermore, this is an exact result for all thresholds $u > 0$. ▲

Example 4.2 For the standard Fréchet model, $F(x) = \exp(-1/x)$, for $x > 0$. Hence,

$$\frac{1 - F(u + y)}{1 - F(u)} = \frac{1 - \exp\{-(u+y)^{-1}\}}{1 - \exp(-u^{-1})} \sim \left(1 + \frac{y}{u}\right)^{-1}$$

as $u \to \infty$, for all $y > 0$. This corresponds to the generalized Pareto distribution with $\xi = 1$ and $\tilde{\sigma} = u$. ▲

Example 4.3 For the uniform distribution model $U(0, 1)$, $F(x) = x$, for $0 \leq x \leq 1$. Hence,

$$\frac{1 - F(u + y)}{1 - F(u)} = \frac{1 - (u + y)}{1 - u} = 1 - \frac{y}{1 - u}$$

for $0 \leq y \leq 1 - u$. This corresponds to the generalized Pareto distribution with $\xi = -1$ and $\tilde{\sigma} = 1 - u$. ▲

Comparison of the limit families obtained here for threshold exceedances with the corresponding block maxima limits obtained in Section 3.1.5 confirms the duality of the two limit model formulations implied by Theorem 4.1. In particular, the values of ξ are common across the two models. Furthermore, the value of $\tilde{\sigma}$ is found to be threshold-dependent, except in the case where the limit model has $\xi = 0$, as implied by Eq. (4.3).

Until this point we have used the notation $\tilde{\sigma}$ to denote the scale parameter of the generalized Pareto distribution, so as to distinguish it from the corresponding parameter of the GEV distribution. For notational convenience we now drop this distinction, using σ to denote the scale parameter within either family.

4.3 Modeling Threshold Excesses

4.3.1 Threshold Selection

Theorem 4.1 suggests the following framework for extreme value modeling. The raw data consist of a sequence of independent and identically distributed measurements $x_1, \ldots, x_n$. Extreme events are identified by defining a high threshold u, for which the exceedances are $\{x_i : x_i > u\}$. Label these exceedances by $x_{(1)}, \ldots, x_{(k)}$, and define threshold excesses by $y_j = x_{(j)} - u$, for $j = 1, \ldots, k$. By Theorem 4.1, the y_j may be regarded as independent realizations of a random variable whose distribution can be approximated by a member of the generalized Pareto family. Inference consists of fitting the generalized Pareto family to the observed threshold exceedances, followed by model verification and extrapolation.

This approach contrasts with the block maxima approach through the characterization of an observation as extreme if it exceeds a high threshold. But the issue of threshold choice is analogous to the choice of block size in the block maxima approach, implying a balance between bias and variance. In this case, too low a threshold is likely to violate the asymptotic basis of the model, leading to bias; too high a threshold will generate few excesses with which the model can be estimated, leading to high variance. The standard practice is to adopt as low a threshold as possible, subject to the limit model providing a reasonable approximation. Two methods are available for this purpose: one is an exploratory technique carried out prior to model estimation; the other is an assessment of the stability of parameter estimates, based on the fitting of models across a range of different thresholds.

In more detail, the first method is based on the mean of the generalized Pareto distribution. If Y has a generalized Pareto distribution with parameters σ and ξ, then

$$\mathrm{E}(Y) = \frac{\sigma}{1-\xi}, \qquad (4.8)$$

4.3 Modeling Threshold Excesses

provided $\xi < 1$. When $\xi \geq 1$ the mean is infinite. Now, suppose the generalized Pareto distribution is valid as a model for the excesses of a threshold u_0 generated by a series $X_1, \ldots, X_n$, of which an arbitrary term is denoted X. By (4.8),

$$\mathrm{E}(X - u_0 \mid X > u_0) = \frac{\sigma_{u_0}}{1 - \xi},$$

provided $\xi < 1$, where we adopt the convention of using σ_{u_0} to denote the scale parameter corresponding to excesses of the threshold u_0. But if the generalized Pareto distribution is valid for excesses of the threshold u_0, it should equally be valid for all thresholds $u > u_0$, subject to the appropriate change of scale parameter to σ_u. Hence, for $u > u_0$,

$$\begin{aligned} \mathrm{E}(X - u \mid X > u) &= \frac{\sigma_u}{1 - \xi} \\ &= \frac{\sigma_{u_0} + \xi u}{1 - \xi} \end{aligned} \quad (4.9)$$

by virtue of (4.3). So, for $u > u_0$, $\mathrm{E}(X - u \mid X > u)$ is a linear function of u. Furthermore, $\mathrm{E}(X - u \mid X > u)$ is simply the mean of the excesses of the threshold u, for which the sample mean of the threshold excesses of u provides an empirical estimate. According to (4.9), these estimates are expected to change linearly with u, at levels of u for which the generalized Pareto model is appropriate. This leads to the following procedure. The locus of points

$$\left\{ \left(u, \frac{1}{n_u} \sum_{i=1}^{n_u} (x_{(i)} - u) \right) : u < x_{\max} \right\},$$

where $x_{(1)}, \ldots, x_{(n_u)}$ consist of the n_u observations that exceed u, and $x_{\max}$ is the largest of the X_i, is termed the **mean residual life plot**. Above a threshold u_0 at which the generalized Pareto distribution provides a valid approximation to the excess distribution, the mean residual life plot should be approximately linear in u. Confidence intervals can be added to the plot based on the approximate normality of sample means.

The interpretation of a mean residual life plot is not always simple in practice. Fig. 4.1 shows the mean residual life plot with approximate 95% confidence intervals for the daily rainfall data of Example 1.6. Once the confidence intervals are taken into account, the graph appears to curve from $u = 0$ to $u \approx 30$, beyond which it is approximately linear until $u \approx 60$, whereupon it decays sharply. It is tempting to conclude that there is no stability until $u = 60$, after which there is approximate linearity. This suggests we take $u_0 = 60$. However, there are just 6 exceedances of the threshold $u = 60$, too few to make meaningful inferences. Moreover, the information in the plot for large values of u is unreliable due to the limited amount of data on which the estimate and confidence interval are based.

80   4. Threshold Models

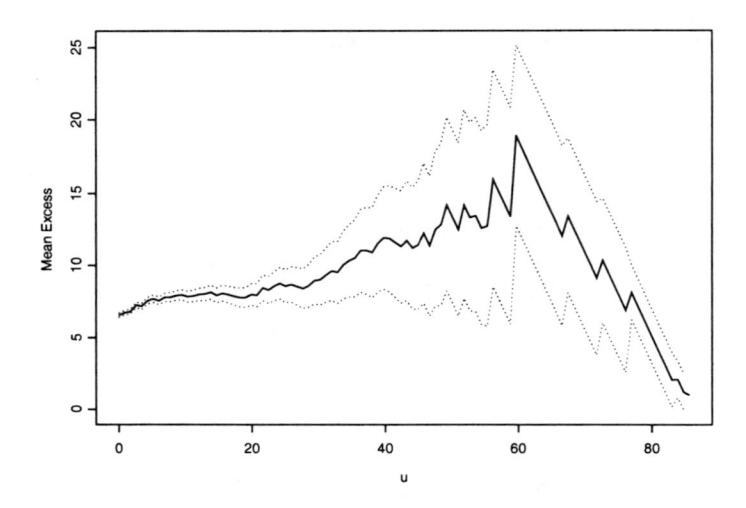

FIGURE 4.1. Mean residual life plot for daily rainfall data.

Accordingly, it is probably better to conclude that there is some evidence for linearity above $u = 30$, and to work initially with a threshold set at $u_0 = 30$.

The second procedure for threshold selection is to estimate the model at a range of thresholds. Above a level u_0 at which the asymptotic motivation for the generalized Pareto distribution is valid, estimates of the shape parameter ξ should be approximately constant, while estimates of σ_u should be linear in u, due to (4.9). We describe this method in greater detail in Section 4.3.4.

4.3.2 Parameter Estimation

Having determined a threshold, the parameters of the generalized Pareto distribution can be estimated by maximum likelihood. Suppose that the values $y_1, \ldots, y_k$ are the k excesses of a threshold u. For $\xi \neq 0$ the log-likelihood is derived from (4.2) as

$$\ell(\sigma, \xi) = -k \log \sigma - (1 + 1/\xi) \sum_{i=1}^{k} \log(1 + \xi y_i/\sigma), \qquad (4.10)$$

provided $(1 + \sigma^{-1} \xi y_i) > 0$ for $i = 1, \ldots, k$; otherwise, $\ell(\sigma, \xi) = -\infty$. In the case $\xi = 0$ the log-likelihood is obtained from (4.4) as

$$\ell(\sigma) = -k \log \sigma - \sigma^{-1} \sum_{i=1}^{k} y_i.$$

Analytical maximization of the log-likelihood is not possible, so numerical techniques are again required, taking care to avoid numerical instabilities when $\xi \approx 0$ in (4.10), and ensuring that the algorithm does not fail due to evaluation outside of the allowable parameter space. Standard errors and confidence intervals for the generalized Pareto distribution are obtained in the usual way from standard likelihood theory.

4.3.3 Return Levels

As discussed in Chapter 3, it is usually more convenient to interpret extreme value models in terms of quantiles or return levels, rather than individual parameter values. So, suppose that a generalized Pareto distribution with parameters σ and ξ is a suitable model for exceedances of a threshold u by a variable X. That is, for $x > u$,

$$\Pr\{X > x \mid X > u\} = \left[1 + \xi \left(\frac{x-u}{\sigma}\right)\right]^{-1/\xi}.$$

It follows that

$$\Pr\{X > x\} = \zeta_u \left[1 + \xi \left(\frac{x-u}{\sigma}\right)\right]^{-1/\xi}, \tag{4.11}$$

where $\zeta_u = \Pr\{X > u\}$. Hence, the level x_m that is exceeded on average once every m observations is the solution of

$$\zeta_u \left[1 + \xi \left(\frac{x_m - u}{\sigma}\right)\right]^{-1/\xi} = \frac{1}{m}. \tag{4.12}$$

Rearranging,

$$x_m = u + \frac{\sigma}{\xi}\left[(m\zeta_u)^\xi - 1\right], \tag{4.13}$$

provided m is sufficiently large to ensure that $x_m > u$. This all assumes that $\xi \neq 0$. If $\xi = 0$, working in the same way with (4.4) leads to

$$x_m = u + \sigma \log(m\zeta_u), \tag{4.14}$$

again provided m is sufficiently large.

By construction, x_m is the **m-observation return level**. From (4.13) and (4.14), plotting x_m against m on a logarithmic scale produces the same qualitative features as return level plots based on the GEV model: linearity if $\xi = 0$; concavity if $\xi > 0$; convexity if $\xi < 0$. For presentation, it is often more convenient to give return levels on an annual scale, so that the N-year return level is the level expected to be exceeded once every N years. If there are n_y observations per year, this corresponds to the m-observation

82   4. Threshold Models

return level, where $m = N \times n_y$. Hence, the N-year return level is defined by

$$z_N = u + \frac{\sigma}{\xi}\left[(Nn_y\zeta_u)^\xi - 1\right],$$

unless $\xi = 0$, in which case

$$z_N = u + \sigma \log(Nn_y\zeta_u).$$

Estimation of return levels requires the substitution of parameter values by their estimates. For σ and ξ this corresponds to substitution by the corresponding maximum likelihood estimates, but an estimate of ζ_u, the probability of an individual observation exceeding the threshold u, is also needed. This has a natural estimator of

$$\hat{\zeta}_u = \frac{k}{n},$$

the sample proportion of points exceeding u. Since the number of exceedances of u follows the binomial $\text{Bin}(n, \zeta_u)$ distribution, $\hat{\zeta}_u$ is also the maximum likelihood estimate of ζ_u.

Standard errors or confidence intervals for x_m can be derived by the delta method, but the uncertainty in the estimate of ζ_u should also be included in the calculation. From standard properties of the binomial distribution, $\text{Var}(\hat{\zeta}_u) \approx \hat{\zeta}_u(1-\hat{\zeta}_u)/n$, so the complete variance-covariance matrix for $(\hat{\zeta}_u, \hat{\sigma}, \hat{\xi})$ is approximately

$$V = \begin{bmatrix} \hat{\zeta}_u(1-\hat{\zeta}_u)/n & 0 & 0 \\ 0 & v_{1,1} & v_{1,2} \\ 0 & v_{2,1} & v_{2,2} \end{bmatrix},$$

where $v_{i,j}$ denotes the (i,j) term of the variance-covariance matrix of $\hat{\sigma}$ and $\hat{\xi}$. Hence, by the delta method,

$$\text{Var}(\hat{x}_m) \approx \nabla x_m^T V \nabla x_m, \tag{4.15}$$

where

$$\nabla x_m^T = \left[\frac{\partial x_m}{\partial \zeta_u}, \frac{\partial x_m}{\partial \sigma}, \frac{\partial x_m}{\partial \xi}\right]$$
$$= \left[\sigma m^\xi \zeta_u^{\xi-1}, \xi^{-1}\left\{(m\zeta_u)^\xi - 1\right\},\right.$$
$$\left. -\sigma\xi^{-2}\left\{(m\zeta_u)^\xi - 1\right\} + \sigma\xi^{-1}(m\zeta_u)^\xi \log(m\zeta_u)\right],$$

evaluated at $(\hat{\zeta}_u, \hat{\sigma}, \hat{\xi})$.

As with previous models, better estimates of precision for parameters and return levels are obtained from the appropriate profile likelihood. For σ or ξ this is straightforward. For return levels, a reparameterization is required. Life is made simpler by ignoring the uncertainty in ζ_u, which is usually small relative to that of the other parameters. From (4.13) and (4.14)

$$\sigma = \begin{cases} \dfrac{(x_m - u)\xi}{(m\zeta_u)^\xi - 1}, & \text{if } \xi \neq 0; \\ \dfrac{x_m - u}{\log(m\zeta_u)}, & \text{if } \xi = 0. \end{cases}$$

With fixed x_m, substitution into (4.10) leads to a one-parameter likelihood that can be maximized with respect to ξ. As a function of x_m, this is the profile log-likelihood for the m-observation return level.

4.3.4 Threshold Choice Revisited

We saw in Section 4.3 that mean residual life plots can be difficult to interpret as a method of threshold selection. A complementary technique is to fit the generalized Pareto distribution at a range of thresholds, and to look for stability of parameter estimates. The argument is as follows.

By Theorem 4.1, if a generalized Pareto distribution is a reasonable model for excesses of a threshold u_0, then excesses of a higher threshold u should also follow a generalized Pareto distribution. The shape parameters of the two distributions are identical. However, denoting by σ_u the value of the generalized Pareto scale parameter for a threshold of $u > u_0$, it follows from (4.3) that

$$\sigma_u = \sigma_{u_0} + \xi(u - u_0), \qquad (4.16)$$

so that the scale parameter changes with u unless $\xi = 0$. This difficulty can be remedied by reparameterizing the generalized Pareto scale parameter as

$$\sigma^* = \sigma_u - \xi u,$$

which is constant with respect to u by virtue of (4.16). Consequently, estimates of both σ^* and ξ should be constant above u_0, if u_0 is a valid threshold for excesses to follow the generalized Pareto distribution. Sampling variability means that the estimates of these quantities will not be exactly constant, but they should be stable after allowance for their sampling errors.

This argument suggests plotting both $\hat{\sigma}^*$ and $\hat{\xi}$ against u, together with confidence intervals for each of these quantities, and selecting u_0 as the lowest value of u for which the estimates remain near-constant. The confidence intervals for $\hat{\xi}$ are obtained immediately from the variance-covariance matrix V. Confidence intervals for $\hat{\sigma}^*$ require the delta method, using

$$\text{Var}(\sigma^*) \approx \nabla\sigma^{*T} V \nabla\sigma^*,$$

where

$$\nabla\sigma^{*T} = \left[\frac{\partial\sigma^*}{\partial\sigma_u}, \frac{\partial\sigma^*}{\partial\xi}\right] = [1, -u].$$

4.3.5 Model Checking

Probability plots, quantile plots, return level plots and density plots are all useful for assessing the quality of a fitted generalized Pareto model. Assuming a threshold u, threshold excesses $y_{(1)} \leq \cdots \leq y_{(k)}$ and an estimated model $\hat{H}$, the probability plot consists of the pairs

$$\{(i/(k+1), \hat{H}(y_{(i)})); \; i = 1, \ldots, k\},$$

where

$$\hat{H}(y) = 1 - \left(1 + \frac{\hat{\xi} y}{\hat{\sigma}}\right)^{-1/\hat{\xi}},$$

provided $\hat{\xi} \neq 0$. If $\hat{\xi} = 0$ the plot is constructed using (4.4) in place of (4.2). Again assuming $\hat{\xi} \neq 0$, the quantile plot consists of the pairs

$$\{(\hat{H}^{-1}(i/(k+1)), y_{(i)}), \; i = 1, \ldots, k\},$$

where

$$\hat{H}^{-1}(y) = u + \frac{\hat{\sigma}}{\hat{\xi}} \left[y^{-\hat{\xi}} - 1\right].$$

If the generalized Pareto model is reasonable for modeling excesses of u, then both the probability and quantile plots should consist of points that are approximately linear.

A return level plot consists of the locus of points $\{(m, \hat{x}_m)\}$ for large values of m, where $\hat{x}_m$ is the estimated m-observation return level:

$$\hat{x}_m = u + \frac{\hat{\sigma}}{\hat{\xi}} \left[(m\hat{\zeta}_u)^{\hat{\xi}} - 1\right],$$

again modified if $\hat{\xi} = 0$. As with the GEV return level plot, it is usual to plot the return level curve on a logarithmic scale to emphasize the effect of extrapolation, and also to add confidence bounds and empirical estimates of the return levels.

Finally, the density function of the fitted generalized Pareto model can be compared to a histogram of the threshold exceedances.

4.4 Examples

4.4.1 Daily Rainfall Data

This example is based on the daily rainfall series discussed in Example 1.6. In Section 4.3 a mean residual life plot for these data suggested a threshold of $u = 30$. Further support for this choice is provided by the model-based check described in Section 4.3.4. The plots of $\hat{\sigma}^*$ and $\hat{\xi}$ against u are shown

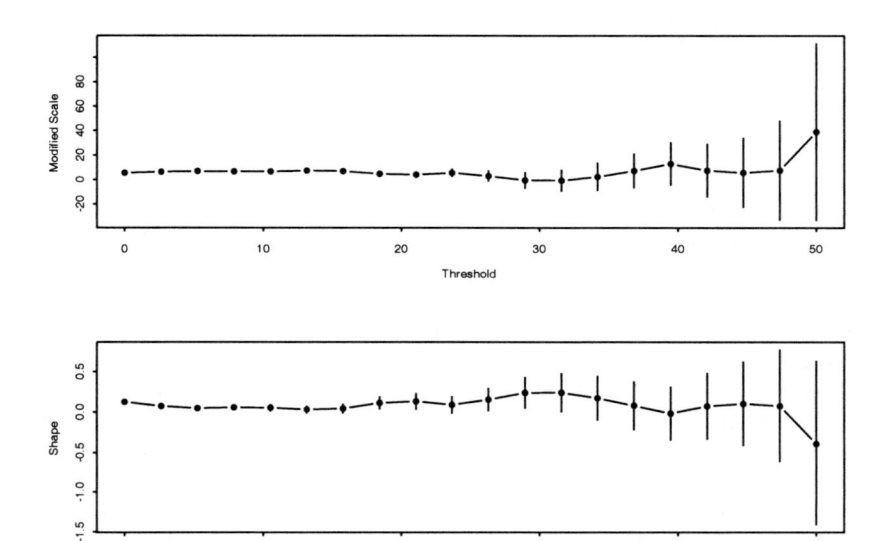

FIGURE 4.2. Parameter estimates against threshold for daily rainfall data.

in Fig. 4.2. The change in pattern for very high thresholds that was observed in the mean residual life plot is also apparent here, but the perturbations are now seen to be small relative to sampling errors. Hence, the selected threshold of $u = 30$ appears reasonable. Maximum likelihood estimates in this case are

$$(\hat{\sigma}, \hat{\xi}) = (7.44, 0.184)$$

with a corresponding maximized log-likelihood of -485.1. The variance-covariance matrix is calculated as

$$\begin{bmatrix} 0.9188 & -0.0655 \\ -0.0655 & 0.0102 \end{bmatrix},$$

leading to standard errors of 0.959 and 0.101 for $\hat{\sigma}$ and $\hat{\xi}$ respectively. In particular, it follows that a 95% confidence interval for ξ is obtained as $0.184 \pm 1.96 \times 0.101 = [-0.014, 0.383]$. The maximum likelihood estimate corresponds, therefore, to an unbounded distribution (since $\hat{\xi} > 0$), and the evidence for this is reasonably strong, since the 95% interval for ξ is almost exclusively in the positive domain.

Since there are 152 exceedances of the threshold $u = 30$ in the complete set of 17531 observations, the maximum likelihood estimate of the exceedance probability is $\hat{\zeta}_u = 152/17531 = 0.00867$, with approximate variance $\mathrm{Var}(\hat{\zeta}_u) = \hat{\zeta}_u(1-\hat{\zeta}_u)/17531 = 4.9 \times 10^{-7}$. Hence, the complete variance-covariance matrix for $(\hat{\zeta}, \hat{\sigma}, \hat{\xi})$ is

$$V = \begin{bmatrix} 4.9 \times 10^{-7} & 0 & 0 \\ 0 & 0.9188 & -0.0655 \\ 0 & -0.0655 & 0.0102 \end{bmatrix}.$$

Since $\hat{\xi} > 0$, it is not useful to carry out a detailed inference of the upper limit. Instead, we focus on extreme return levels. The data are daily, so the 100-year return level corresponds to the m-observation return level with $m = 365 \times 100$. Substitution into (4.13) and (4.15) gives $\hat{x}_m = 106.3$ and $\mathrm{Var}(\hat{x}_m) = 431.3$, leading to a 95% confidence interval for x_m of $106.3 \pm 1.96\sqrt{431.3} = [65.6, 147.0]$.

Comparison with the observed data casts some doubt on the accuracy of this interval: in the 48 years of observation, the lower interval limit of 65.6 was exceeded 6 times, suggesting that the 100-year return level is almost certainly not as low in value as the confidence interval implies is plausible. Better accuracy is achieved by using profile likelihood intervals. Fig. 4.3 shows the profile log-likelihood for ξ in this example. By Theorem 2.6 an approximate 95% confidence interval for ξ is obtained from this graph as $[0.019, 0.418]$. This is not so different from the previous interval obtained previously, but strengthens slightly the conclusion that $\xi > 0$. The profile log-likelihood for the 100-year return level is plotted in Fig. 4.4. In this case the surface is highly asymmetric, reflecting the greater uncertainty about large values of the process. The 95% confidence interval for the 100-year return level is obtained from the profile log-likelihood as $[81.6, 185.7]$, an interval which now excludes the implausible range that formed part of the interval based on the delta method. Furthermore, the upper limit of 185.7 is very much greater than the delta-method value, more realistically accounting for the genuine uncertainties of extreme model extrapolation. This again illustrates that intervals derived from the delta method are anti-conservative, and should be replaced by profile likelihood intervals whenever a more precise measure of uncertainty is required.

Finally, diagnostic plots for the fitted generalized Pareto model are shown in Fig. 4.5. None of the plots gives any real cause for concern about the quality of the fitted model.

4.4.2 Dow Jones Index Series

The Dow Jones Index data discussed in Example 1.8 provide a second example for exploring the utility of the threshold exceedance modeling approach. Because of the strong non-stationarity observed in the original series $X_1, \ldots, X_n$, the data are transformed as $\tilde{X}_i = \log X_i - \log X_{i-1}$. Fig. 1.9 suggests that the transformed series is reasonably close to stationarity.

4.4 Examples   87

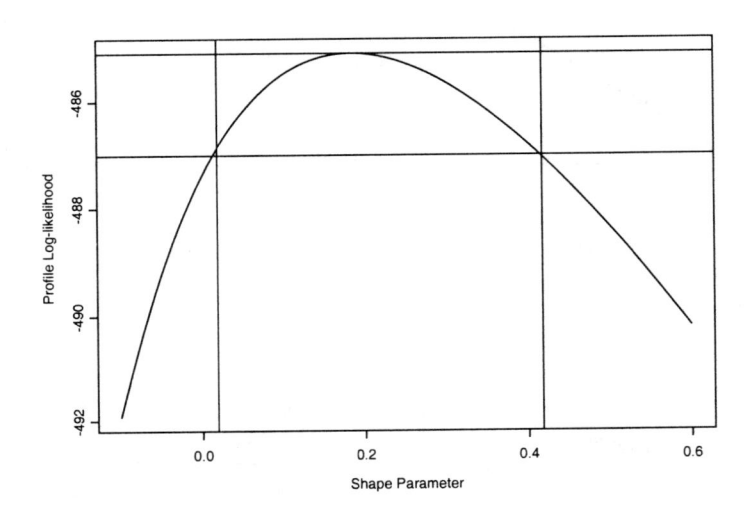

FIGURE 4.3. Profile likelihood for ξ in threshold excess model of daily rainfall data.

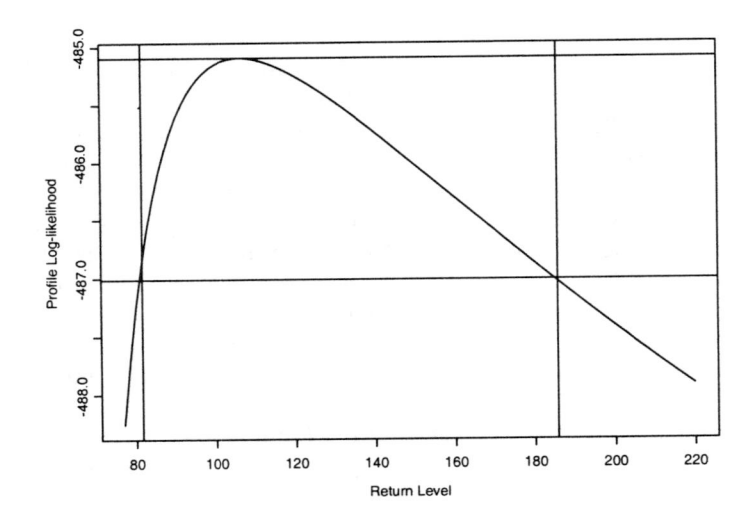

FIGURE 4.4. Profile likelihood for 100-year return level in threshold excess model of daily rainfall data.

88   4. Threshold Models

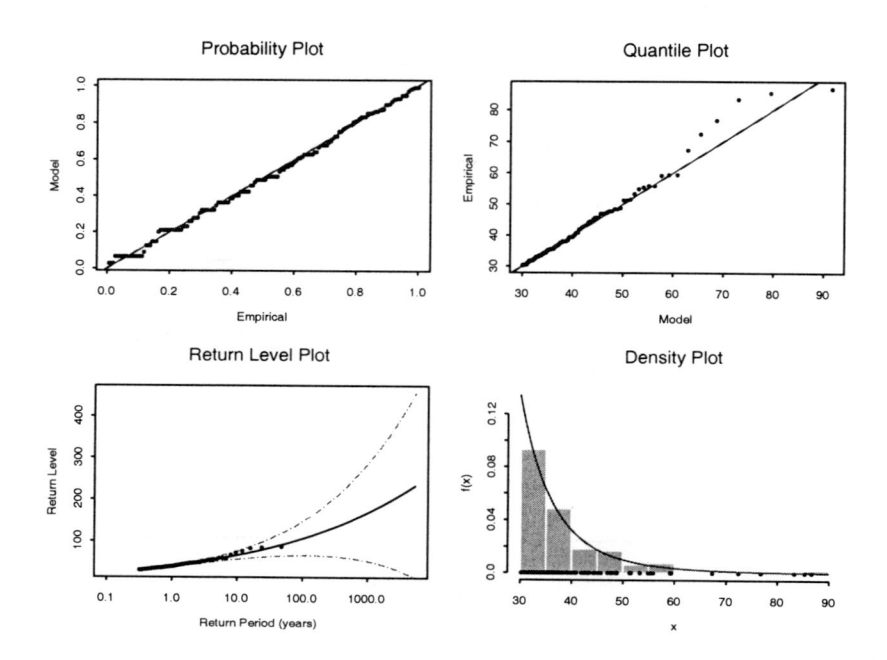

FIGURE 4.5. Diagnostic plots for threshold excess model fitted to daily rainfall data.

For convenience of presentation, the data are now re-scaled as $\tilde{X} \to 100\tilde{X}$. A mean residual life for the resulting $\tilde{X}_i$ series is shown in Fig. 4.6. The plot is initially linear, but shows substantial curvature in the range $-1 \leq u \leq 2$. For $u > 2$ the plot is reasonably linear when judged relative to confidence intervals, suggesting we set $u = 2$. This choice leads to 37 exceedances in the series of length 1303, so $\hat{\zeta}_u = 37/1303 = 0.028$. The maximum likelihood estimates of the generalized Pareto distribution parameters are $(\hat{\sigma}, \hat{\xi}) = (0.495, 0.288)$, with standard errors of 0.150 and 0.258 respectively. The maximum likelihood estimate corresponds, therefore, to an unbounded excess distribution, though the evidence for this is not overwhelming: 0 lies comfortably inside a 95% confidence interval for ξ.

Diagnostic plots for the fitted generalized Pareto distribution are shown in Fig. 4.7. The goodness-of-fit in the quantile plot seems unconvincing, but the confidence intervals on the return level plot suggest that the model departures are not large after allowance for sampling. The return level plot also illustrates the very large uncertainties that accrue once the model is extrapolated to higher levels.

In the context of financial modeling, extreme quantiles of the daily returns are generally referred to as the **value-at-risk**. It follows that the

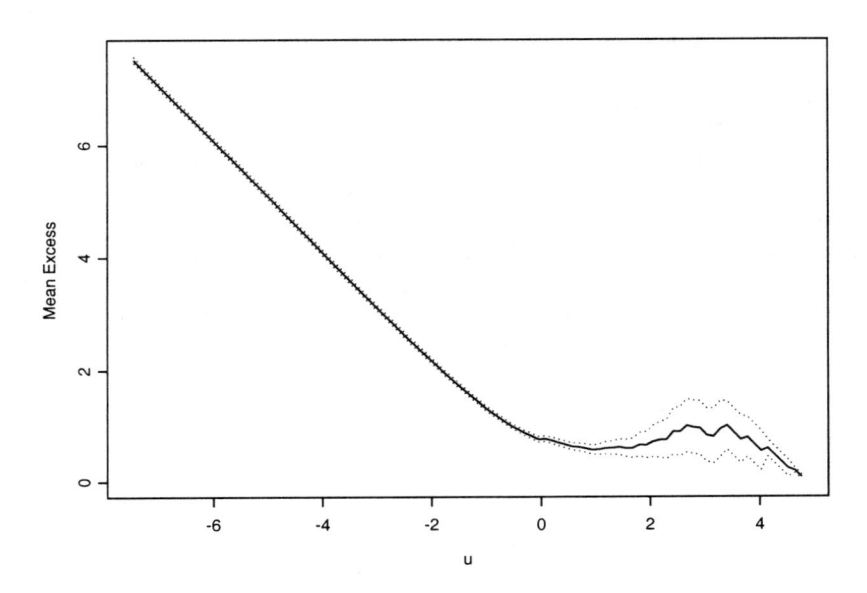

FIGURE 4.6. Mean residual life plot for transformed Dow Jones Index data.

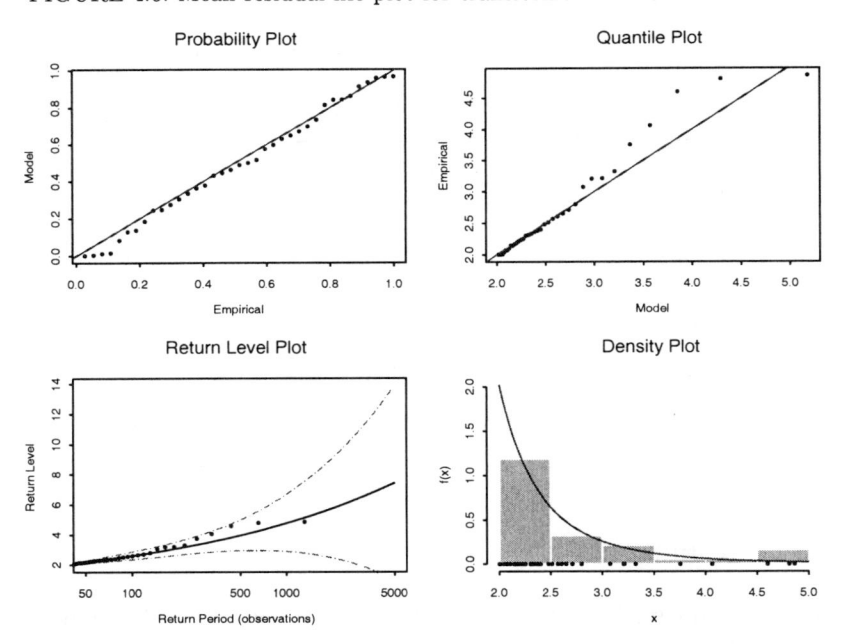

FIGURE 4.7. Diagnostic plots for threshold excess model fitted to transformed Dow Jones Index data.

generalized Pareto threshold model provides a direct method for the estimation of value-at-risk. Furthermore, the return level plot is simply a graph of value-at-risk against risk, on a convenient scale.

Finally, we discussed in the introduction of Example 1.8 that financial series often have a rich structure of temporal dependence. The transformation $X_i \to \tilde{X}_i$ is successful in reducing non-stationarity – the pattern of variation is approximately constant through time – but the induced series is not independent. That is, the distribution of $\tilde{X}_i$ is dependent on the history of the process $\{\tilde{X}_1, \ldots, \tilde{X}_{i-1}\}$. One illustration of this is provided by Fig. 4.8, which shows the threshold exceedances at their times of occurrence. If the series were independent the times of threshold exceedances would be uniform distributed; in actual fact the data of Fig. 4.8 demonstrate a tendency for the extreme events to cluster together. Such violation of the assumptions of Theorem 4.1 brings into doubt the validity of the simple threshold excess model for the Dow Jones Index series. We return to this issue in Chapter 5.

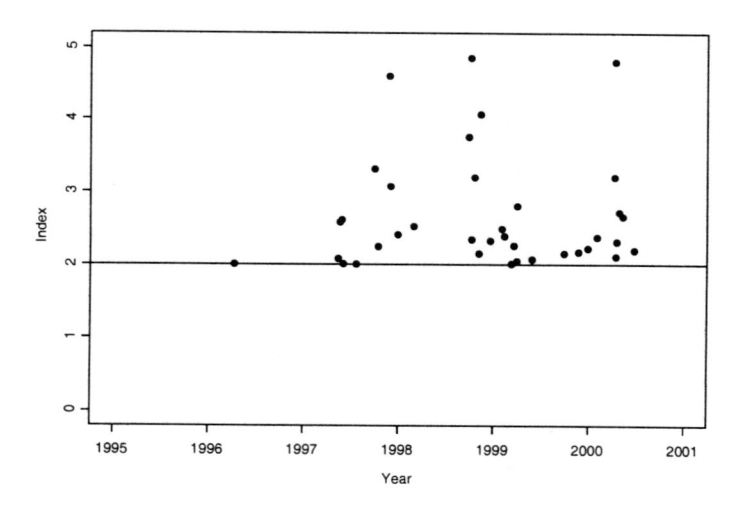

FIGURE 4.8. Threshold exceedances by transformed Dow Jones Index series.

4.5 Further Reading

The basic strategy of modeling threshold excesses has a long history in the hydrological literature, though the excesses were originally assumed to have a distribution belonging to the family of exponential distributions rather than the complete generalized Pareto family. The arguments leading to the generalized Pareto model are attributable to Pickands (1975).

Statistical properties of the threshold approach were looked at in detail by Davison & Smith (1990), synthesizing earlier work in Davison (1984) and Smith (1984). In particular, they advocated the use of the mean residual life plot for threshold selection, and a likelihood approach to inference. Applications of the threshold approach are now widespread: see, for example, Grady (1992), Walshaw (1994) and Fitzgerald (1989).

A popular alternative to maximum likelihood estimation in the threshold excess model is a class of procedures based on functions of order statistics. These techniques often have an interpretation in terms of properties of quantile plots on appropriate scales, and generally incorporate procedures for threshold selection. Many of the techniques are variants on a proposal by Hill (1975); Dekkers & de Haan (1993), Beirlant et al. (1996) and Drees et al. (2000) make modified suggestions.

5
Extremes of Dependent Sequences

5.1 Introduction

Each of the extreme value models derived so far has been obtained through mathematical arguments that assume an underlying process consisting of a sequence of independent random variables. However, for the types of data to which extreme value models are commonly applied, temporal independence is usually an unrealistic assumption. In particular, extreme conditions often persist over several consecutive observations, bringing into question the appropriateness of models such as the GEV. A detailed investigation of this question requires a mathematical treatment at a greater level of sophistication than we have adopted so far. However, the basic ideas are not difficult and the main result has a simple heuristic interpretation. A more precise development is given by Leadbetter et al. (1983).

The most natural generalization of a sequence of independent random variables is to a stationary series. Stationarity, which is a more realistic assumption for many physical processes, corresponds to a series whose variables may be mutually dependent, but whose stochastic properties are homogeneous through time. So, for example, if $X_1, X_2, \ldots$ is a stationary series, then X_1 must have the same distribution as X_{101}, and the joint distribution of (X_1, X_2) must be the same as that of (X_{101}, X_{102}), though X_1 need not be independent of X_2 or X_{102}.

Dependence in stationary series can take many different forms, and it is impossible to develop a general characterization of the behavior of extremes unless some constraints are imposed. With practical applications in mind, it is usual to assume a condition that limits the extent of long-range dependence at extreme levels, so that the events $X_i > u$ and $X_j > u$ are approximately independent, provided u is high enough, and time points i and j have a large separation. In other words, extreme events are close to independent at times that are far enough apart. Many stationary series satisfy this property. More importantly, it is a property that is often plausible for physical processes. For example, knowledge that it rained heavily today might influence the probability of extreme rainfall in one or two days' time, but not for a specified day in, say, three months' time.

Eliminating long-range dependence at extreme levels in this way focuses attention on the effect of short-range dependence. Our heuristic arguments below, which mirror the more precise mathematical formulations, lead to a simple quantification of such effects on the standard extreme value limits.

5.2 Maxima of Stationary Sequences

The first step is to formulate a condition that makes precise the notion of extreme events being near-independent if they are sufficiently distant in time.

Definition 5.1 A stationary series $X_1, X_2, \ldots$ is said to satisfy the $D(u_n)$ condition if, for all $i_1 < \ldots < i_p < j_1 < \ldots < j_q$ with $j_1 - i_p > l$,

$$\left| \Pr\{X_{i_1} \leq u_n, \ldots, X_{i_p} \leq u_n, X_{j_1} \leq u_n, \ldots, X_{j_q} \leq u_n\} \right.$$
$$\left. - \Pr\{X_{i_1} \leq u_n, \ldots, X_{i_p} \leq u_n\} \Pr\{X_{j_1} \leq u_n, \ldots, X_{j_q} \leq u_n\} \right| \leq \alpha(n, l),$$
(5.1)

where $\alpha(n, l_n) \to 0$ for some sequence l_n such that $l_n/n \to 0$ as $n \to \infty$. △

For sequences of independent variables, the difference in probabilities expressed in (5.1) is exactly zero for *any* sequence u_n. More generally, we will require that the $D(u_n)$ condition holds only for a specific sequence of thresholds u_n that increases with n. For such a sequence, the $D(u_n)$ condition ensures that, for sets of variables that are far enough apart, the difference of probabilities expressed in (5.1), while not zero, is sufficiently close to zero to have no effect on the limit laws for extremes. This is summarized by the following result.

Theorem 5.1 Let $X_1, X_2 \ldots$ be a stationary process and define $M_n = \max\{X_1, \ldots, X_n\}$. Then if $\{a_n > 0\}$ and $\{b_n\}$ are sequences of constants such that

$$\Pr\{(M_n - b_n)/a_n \leq z\} \to G(z),$$

where G is a non-degenerate distribution function, and the $D(u_n)$ condition is satisfied with $u_n = a_n z + b_n$ for every real z, G is a member of the generalized extreme value family of distributions. □

The proof of this result is similar to that of Theorem 3.1, but extra care is needed to demonstrate that the $D(u_n)$ condition with $u_n = a_n x + b_n$ is sufficient for the effects of dependence in the series to have no influence on the limit result. The result is remarkable since it implies that, provided a series has limited long-range dependence at extreme levels (in the sense that the $D(u_n)$ condition makes precise), maxima of stationary series follow the same distributional limit laws as those of independent series. However, the parameters of the limit distribution are affected by the dependence in the series. We can examine this by comparing the distributions of the maxima of a stationary series and of a series of independent variables having the same marginal distribution. We let $X_1, X_2, \ldots$ be a stationary series with marginal distribution function F, and define an associated series $X_1^*, X_2^* \ldots$ of *independent* random variables, such that each of the X_i^* also has distribution function F. In particular, we compare the limiting distributions of $M_n = \max\{X_1, \ldots, X_n\}$ and $M_n^* = \max\{X_1^*, \ldots, X_n^*\}$ as $n \to \infty$. Since the marginal distributions of the X_i and X_i^* series are the same, any difference in the limiting distributions of maxima must be attributable to dependence in the $\{X_i\}$ series.

Before discussing the general result, it is instructive to consider an example.

Example 5.1 Let $Y_0, Y_1, Y_2, \ldots$ be an independent sequence of random variables with distribution function

$$F_Y(y) = \exp\left\{-\frac{1}{(a+1)y}\right\}, \quad y > 0,$$

where $0 \leq a \leq 1$ is a parameter. Now define the process X_i by

$$X_0 = Y_0, \quad X_i = \max\{aY_{i-1}, Y_i\}, \quad i = 1, \ldots, n.$$

For each $i = 1, \ldots, n$,

$$\Pr\{X_i \leq x\} = \Pr\{aY_{i-1} \leq x, \, Y_i \leq x\} = \exp(-1/x),$$

provided $x > 0$. Hence, the marginal distribution of the X_i series, for $i = 1, 2, \ldots$, is standard Fréchet. It is also easy to check that the series is stationary. Now, let $X_1^*, X_2^*, \ldots$ be a series of independent variables having a marginal standard Fréchet distribution, and define $M_n^* = \max\{X_1^*, \ldots, X_n^*\}$. Then,

$$\Pr\{M_n^* \leq nz\} = [\exp\{-1/(nz)\}]^n = \exp(-1/z).$$

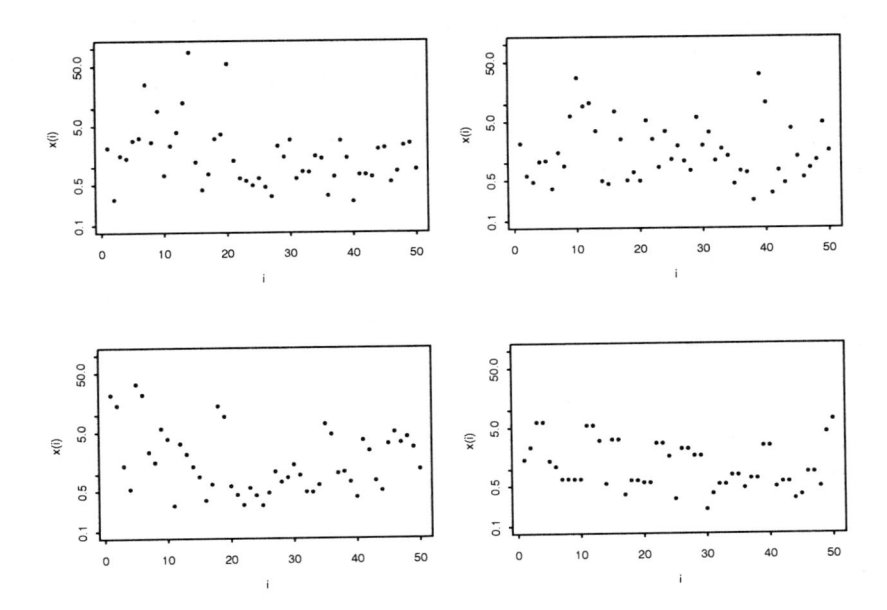

FIGURE 5.1. Simulated series for different values of parameter a in Example 5.1: top left, $a = 0$; top right, $a = 1/3$; bottom left, $a = 2/3$; bottom right, $a = 1$

On the other hand, for $M_n = \max\{X_1, \ldots, X_n\}$,

$$\begin{aligned}
\Pr\{M_n \leq nz\} &= \Pr\{X_1 \leq nz, \ldots, X_n \leq nz\} \\
&= \Pr\{Y_1 \leq nz, aY_1 \leq nz, \ldots, aY_{n-1} \leq nz, Y_n \leq nz\} \\
&= \Pr\{Y_1 \leq nz, \ldots, Y_n \leq nz\} \\
&= \left[\exp\left\{-\frac{1}{(a+1)nz}\right\}\right]^n \\
&= \{\exp(-1/z)\}^{\frac{1}{a+1}},
\end{aligned}$$

where we have used the fact that $a \leq 1$. It follows, in particular, that

$$\Pr\{M_n^* \leq nz\} = [\Pr\{M_n \leq nz\}]^{\frac{1}{a+1}} \tag{5.2}$$

▲

Further insight is gained by looking at simulated sequences of the stationary series in Example 5.1 for different values of the parameter a. Figure 5.1 shows plots of such series on a logarithmic scale for $a = 0, 1/3, 2/3$ and 1 respectively. The marginal distribution of each series is the same but, with increasing a, there is a tendency for extreme values to occur in groups. In particular, when $a = 1$, the largest observations invariably occur in pairs. Though obscured by sampling variability, it also follows that the maximum over the 50 observations has a tendency to decrease as a increases. This is inevitable because of the relationship between M_n and M_n^* derived in (5.2).

A similar linkage between the distributions of M_n and M_n^* to that in Example 5.1 can be shown to hold, under suitable regularity conditions, for a wide class of stationary processes. A summary of the result is given in Theorem 5.2.

Theorem 5.2 Let $X_1, X_2, \ldots$ be a stationary process and $X_1^*, X_2^*, \ldots$ be a sequence of independent variables with the same marginal distribution. Define $M_n = \max\{X_1, \ldots, X_n\}$ and $M_n^* = \max\{X_1^*, \ldots, X_n^*\}$. Under suitable regularity conditions,

$$\Pr\{(M_n^* - b_n)/a_n \leq z\} \to G_1(z)$$

as $n \to \infty$ for normalizing sequences $\{a_n > 0\}$ and $\{b_n\}$, where G_1 is a non-degenerate distribution function, if and only if

$$\Pr\{(M_n - b_n)/a_n \leq z\} \to G_2(z),$$

where

$$G_2(z) = G_1^\theta(z) \tag{5.3}$$

for a constant θ such that $0 < \theta \leq 1$. □

Theorem 5.2 implies that if maxima of a stationary series converge – which, by Theorem 5.1 they will do, provided an appropriate $D(u_n)$ condition is satisfied – the limit distribution is related to the limit distribution of an independent series according to Eq. (5.3). The effect of dependence in the stationary series is simply a replacement of G_1 as the limit distribution – which would have arisen for the associated independent series with same marginal distribution – with G_1^θ. This is consistent with Theorem 5.1, because if G_1 is a GEV distribution, so is G_1^θ. More precisely, if G_1 corresponds to the GEV distribution with parameters (μ, σ, ξ), and $\xi \neq 0$, then

$$\begin{aligned}
G_1^\theta(z) &= \exp\left\{-\left[1 + \xi\left(\frac{z-\mu}{\sigma}\right)\right]^{-1/\xi}\right\}^\theta \\
&= \exp\left\{-\theta\left[1 + \xi\left(\frac{z-\mu}{\sigma}\right)\right]^{-1/\xi}\right\} \\
&= \exp\left\{-\left[1 + \xi\left(\frac{z-\mu^*}{\sigma^*}\right)\right]^{-1/\xi}\right\}
\end{aligned}$$

where

$$\mu^* = \mu - \frac{\sigma}{\xi}(1 - \theta^{-\xi}) \quad \text{and} \quad \sigma^* = \sigma\theta^\xi.$$

Accordingly, if the approximate distribution of M_n^* is GEV with parameters (μ, σ, ξ), the approximate distribution of M_n is GEV with parameters (μ^*, σ^*, ξ). In particular, the shape parameters of the two distributions are equal. Similarly, if G_1 corresponds to the Gumbel distribution with location and scale parameters μ and σ respectively, G_2 is also a Gumbel distribution, with parameters

$$\mu^* = \mu + \sigma \log \theta \quad \text{and} \quad \sigma^* = \sigma.$$

The quantity θ defined by (5.3) is termed the **extremal index**. A more precise statement of Theorem 5.2, together with proofs, is given in Chapter 3 of Leadbetter et al. (1983). In particular, the various regularity conditions required to establish the result can be found there. Furthermore, the definition of the extremal index can be extended to include the case $\theta = 0$, though in this case the result of Theorem 5.2 does not hold true.

Looking back at Example 5.1, the extremal index is $\theta = (a+1)^{-1}$ for the stationary process defined there. Another way of interpreting the extremal index of a stationary series is in terms of the propensity of the process to cluster at extreme levels. Loosely,

$$\theta = (\text{limiting mean cluster size})^{-1}, \qquad (5.4)$$

where limiting is in the sense of clusters of exceedances of increasingly high thresholds. For example, in the $a = 1$ case of Example 5.1, $\theta = 0.5$, consistent by (5.4) with a mean cluster size of 2, which seems apparent from Figure 5.1.

Finally, we remark that for independent series, the extremal index $\theta = 1$. This is obvious from Theorem 5.2 as $\{X_i\}$ and $\{X_i^*\}$ comprise the same series. The converse, however, is not true: there are many stationary series with $\theta = 1$ that are not a series of independent observations. Indeed, it is easy to construct processes for which the dependence between successive observations, as measured by the correlation coefficient ρ, is arbitrarily close to 1, but for which θ is also equal to 1. This means that special consideration has to be given to the issue of dependence at extreme levels of a series. It also means that care is needed when using the asymptotic theory of extremes: a series for which $\theta = 1$ means that dependence is negligible at *asymptotically high* levels, but not necessarily so at extreme levels that are relevant for any particular application.

5.3 Modeling Stationary Series

Theorems 5.1 and 5.2 are equivalents of the asymptotic laws for maxima obtained in earlier chapters. But what effect should such results have on extreme value modeling of stationary series in practice?

5.3.1 Models for Block Maxima

For block maxima data the answer is particularly simple. Provided long-range dependence at extreme levels is weak, so that the data can be reasonably considered as a realization of a process satisfying an appropriate $D(u_n)$ condition, the distribution of the block maximum falls within the same family of distributions as would be appropriate if the series were independent. So, for example, it is still appropriate to model the distribution of the annual maximum using the GEV family using the methods discussed in Chapter 3. The parameters themselves are different from those that would have been obtained had the series been independent, but since the parameters are to be estimated anyway, this is unimportant. The conclusion is that dependence in data can be ignored, so far as the modeling of block maxima is concerned.

This argument substantially strengthens the case for using the GEV family as a model for annual maxima. Many of the original objections to the use of asymptotic models for extreme value analysis were based on the argument that the assumptions on which such models were derived are implausible for genuine physical processes. But, the relaxation from independent series to stationary series goes a long way to removing such concerns. An unresolved aspect of the arguments, however, concerns the validity of the limiting results as approximations. The basic premise is that the limiting distribution of M_n can be used as an approximation for large, finite n. With stationary series, as we have seen, M_n has similar statistical properties to $M_{n\theta}^*$, corresponding to the maximum over $n\theta$ observations of an independent series. But in reducing from n to $n\theta$ the effective number of observations, the quality of the approximation is diminished. So, although the limiting result is the same for stationary and independent series, the accuracy of the GEV family as an approximation to the distribution of block maxima is likely to diminish with increased levels of dependence in the series.

5.3.2 Threshold Models

Just as the GEV remains an appropriate model for block maxima of stationary series, similar arguments suggest that the generalized Pareto distribution remains appropriate for threshold excesses. However, the fact that extremes may have a tendency to cluster in a stationary series means that some change of practice is needed. The assumption made in Chapter 4 was that individual excesses were independent, leading to the log-likelihood (4.10). For stationary series, the usual asymptotic arguments imply that the marginal distribution of excesses of a high threshold is generalized Pareto, but they do not lead to a specification of the joint distribution of neighboring excesses.

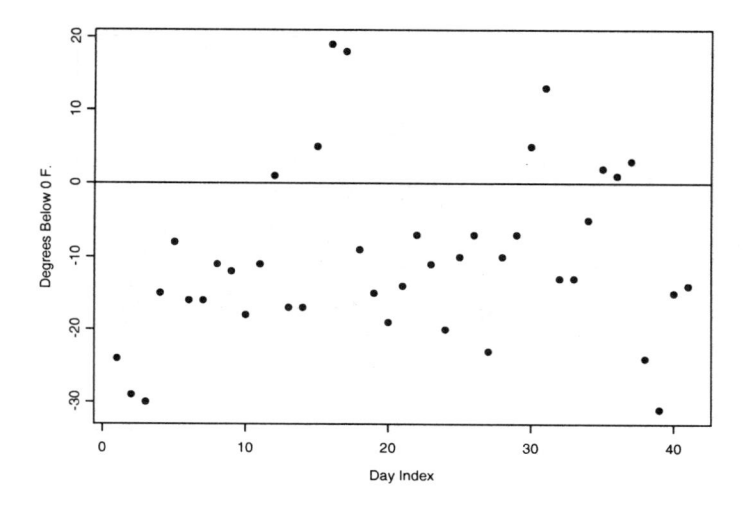

FIGURE 5.2. Portion of Wooster daily minimum temperature series.

To consider this issue in the context of an application, Figure 5.2 shows a section of the Wooster daily minimum temperature series that is approximately stationary. The data have been negated, so large values correspond to extremely cold temperatures. A threshold of zero degrees Fahrenheit has also been added. Threshold exceedances are seen to occur in groups, implying that one extremely cold day is likely to be followed by another. The asymptotics suggest that the distribution of any one of the threshold excesses might be modeled using the generalized Pareto distribution, but the clustering induces dependence in the observations, invalidating the log-likelihood (4.10). Moreover, there is no general theory to provide an alternative likelihood that incorporates the dependence in the observations.

Various suggestions, with different degrees of sophistication, have been made for dealing with the problem of dependent exceedances in the threshold exceedance model. The most widely-adopted method is **declustering**, which corresponds to a filtering of the dependent observations to obtain a set of threshold excesses that are approximately independent. This works by:

1. using an empirical rule to define clusters of exceedances;

2. identifying the maximum excess within each cluster;

3. assuming cluster maxima to be independent, with conditional excess distribution given by the generalized Pareto distribution;

4. fitting the generalized Pareto distribution to the cluster maxima.

100   5. Extremes of Dependent Sequences

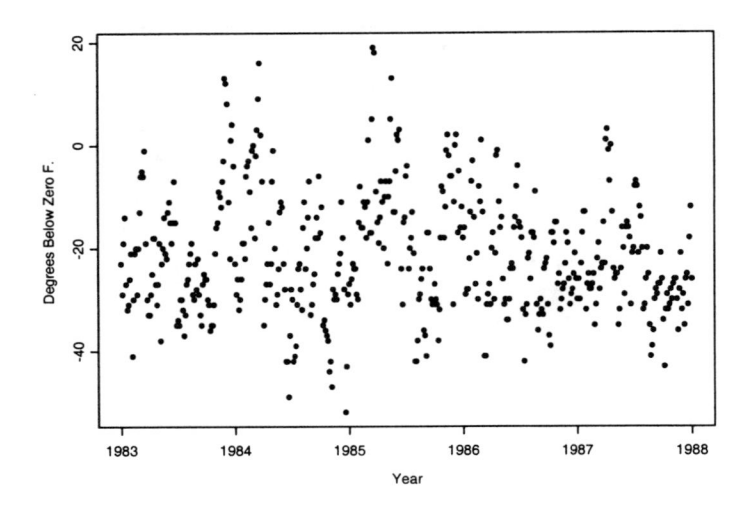

FIGURE 5.3. Wooster daily minimum temperatures (winters only).

The method is simple, but has its limitations. In particular, results can be sensitive to the arbitrary choices made in cluster determination and there is arguably a wastage of information in discarding all data except the cluster maxima.

5.3.3   Wooster Temperature Series

To illustrate the declustering method, we look in some detail at the Wooster minimum daily temperature series, restricting attention to the November–February winter months. For the five-year observation period this series is shown in Fig. 5.3. Though there is still some evidence of non-stationarity, it is considerably weaker than in the entire series.

A simple way of determining clusters of extremes is to specify a threshold u, and define consecutive exceedances of u to belong to the same cluster. Once we obtain an observation that falls below u, the cluster is deemed to have terminated. The next exceedance of u then initiates the next cluster. However, this allows separate clusters to be separated by a single observation, in which case the argument for independence across cluster maxima is flimsy. Furthermore, the separation of extreme events into clusters is likely to be sensitive to the particular choice of threshold. To overcome these deficiencies it is more common to consider a cluster to be active until r consecutive values fall below the threshold for some pre-specified value of r. The choice of r requires care: too small a value will lead to the problem of independence being unrealistic for nearby clusters; too large a value will

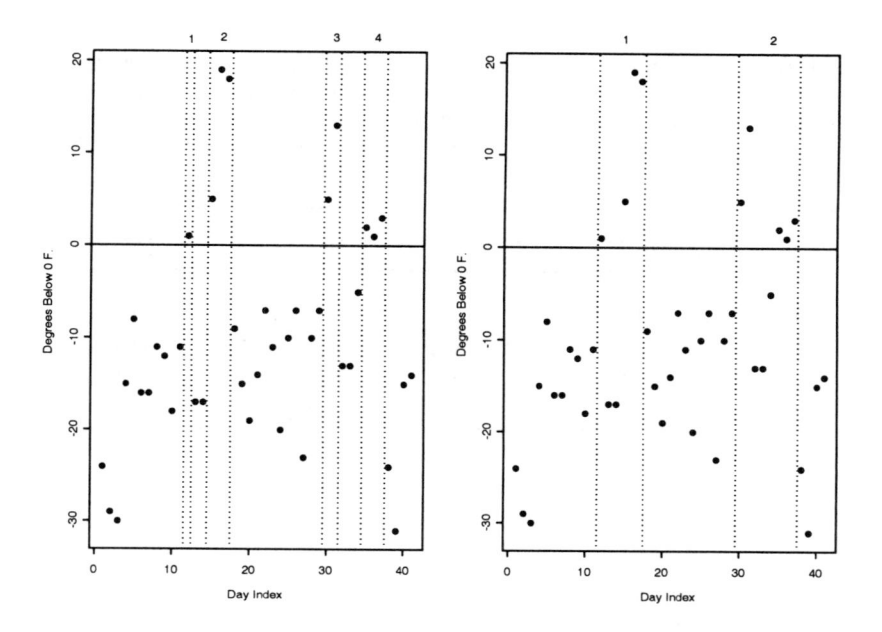

FIGURE 5.4. Portion of Wooster daily minimum temperature series with two possible cluster groupings.

lead to a concatenation of clusters that could reasonably have been considered as independent, and therefore to a loss of valuable data. As we have encountered several times, the issue is a trade-off between bias and variance, for which there are no general guidelines. In the absence of anything more formal, it is usual to rely on common-sense judgement, but also to check the sensitivity of results to the choice of r.

For the section of data shown in Fig. 5.2, the effect of different choices for r on cluster identification is shown in Fig. 5.4. With $r = 1$ or $r = 2$ four clusters are obtained; with $r = 3$ just two clusters are obtained. Working with the entire winter series, maximum likelihood estimates for various combinations of threshold, u, and minimum gap between clusters, r, are shown in Table 5.1.

Assessment is not straightforward because the generalized Pareto distribution involves two parameters, and the value of the scale parameter is expected to change with threshold. However, the shape parameter estimates appear stable with respect to both threshold choice and the choice of r. Standard errors also decrease with both u and r, since either change leads to an increase in the amount of data being modeled.

A clearer impression of model stability is obtained from return levels. Since the rate at which clusters occur, rather than the rate of individual

102   5. Extremes of Dependent Sequences

TABLE 5.1. Estimated features of threshold model fitted to negated Wooster temperature series (winters only) with threshold u and minimum gap r between clusters. The terms $\hat{\sigma}$ and $\hat{\xi}$ correspond to generalized Pareto distribution estimates; $\hat{x}_{100}$ corresponds to the 100-year return level; $\hat{\theta}$ corresponds to the extremal index. Figures in parentheses are standard errors.

	$u = -10$		$u = -20$	
	$r = 2$	$r = 4$	$r = 2$	$r = 4$
n_c	31	20	43	29
$\hat{\sigma}$	11.8 (3.0)	14.2 (5.2)	17.4 (3.6)	19.0 (4.9)
$\hat{\xi}$	−0.29 (0.19)	−0.38 (0.30)	−0.36 (0.15)	−0.41 (0.19)
$\hat{x}_{100}$	27.7 (12.0)	26.6 (14.4)	26.2 (9.3)	25.7 (9.9)
$\hat{\theta}$	0.42	0.27	0.24	0.16

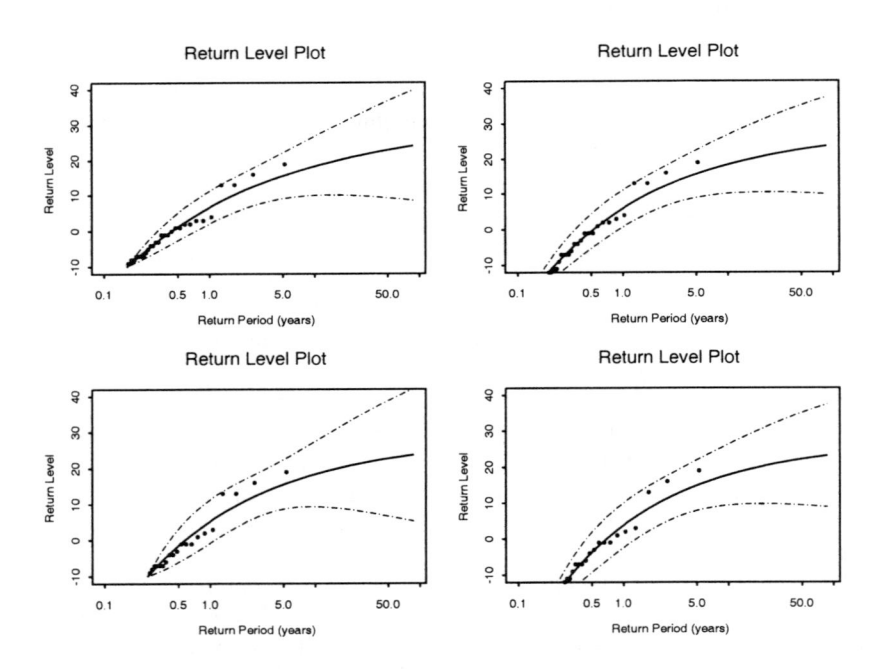

FIGURE 5.5. Return level plots for Wooster daily minimum temperature series based on different threshold and cluster definitions: top left, $u = -10, r = 2$; top right, $u = -10, r = 4$; bottom left, $u = -20, r = 2$; bottom right, $u = -20, r = 4$.

exceedances, must be taken into account, the m-observation return level is

$$x_m = u + \frac{\sigma}{\xi}\left[(m\zeta_u\theta)^\xi - 1\right], \tag{5.5}$$

where σ and ξ are the parameters of the threshold excess generalized Pareto distribution, ζ_u is the probability of an exceedance of u, and θ is the extremal index. Denoting the number of exceedances of the threshold u by n_u, and the number of clusters obtained above u by n_c, ζ_u and θ_u are estimated as

$$\hat{\zeta}_u = \frac{n_u}{n} \quad \text{and} \quad \hat{\theta} = \frac{n_c}{n_u}.$$

It follows that the component $\zeta_u\theta$ in Eq. (5.5) can be estimated by n_c/n. Estimates of θ for the Wooster winter temperature series are included in Table 5.1. Being empirical, they are seen to be sensitive to the choice of u and r. Estimates of the 100-year return level, together with standard errors, are also included in Table 5.1. These values are similar across all choices of u and r, suggesting that inference on return levels is robust despite the subjective choices that need to be made. In particular, the apparent instability in the extremal index estimate appears not to impact unduly on the return level estimation. These observations are confirmed by the stability in the estimated return level curves shown in Fig. 5.5.

5.3.4 Dow Jones Index Series

We conclude this chapter by returning briefly to the Dow Jones Index data introduced in Example 1.8. Using a declustering scheme with $r = 4$ and a threshold of $u = 2$ (after the data have been re-scaled by a factor of 100) leads to generalized Pareto distribution parameter estimates $\hat{\sigma} = 0.538$ (0.177) and $\hat{\xi} = 0.270$ (0.281), with standard errors given in parentheses. The extremal index for the series is estimated as $\hat{\theta} = 0.865$, suggesting only weak dependence at extreme levels.

A return level plot for the fitted model is shown in Fig. 5.6. This takes into account both the marginal features of extremes of the series through the generalized Pareto distribution parameter estimates, and dependence at extreme levels of the series through the extremal index estimate. As discussed in Chapter 4, for financial series a return level plot can also be regarded as a plot of value-at-risk against risk. The agreement in Fig. 5.6 of empirical and model-based estimates suggests the fitted model is working well. The large confidence intervals that are obtained for extreme return levels reflect the fact that there is little information with which to make future predictions with any degree of certainty.

104   5. Extremes of Dependent Sequences

Return Level Plot

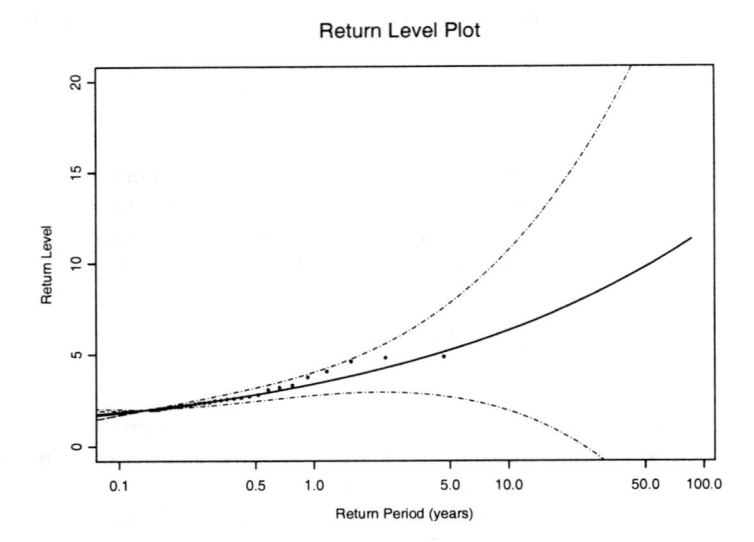

FIGURE 5.6. Return level plot for log-daily returns of Dow Jones Index series.

5.4 Further Reading

The general characterization of extremes of stationary processes dates back to the 1970's. The work of Leadbetter (1983) was instrumental in unifying these results, and developing a characterization that was broadly applicable with only weak regularity conditions. Leadbetter et al. (1983) give a detailed account of the whole development. Extremal properties of special classes of stationary sequences have also been studied: see, for example, O'Brien (1987), Smith (1992) and Perfekt (1994) for the extremal properties of Markov chains; Rootzén (1986) for moving average processes; de Haan et al. (1989) for ARCH processes; and Leadbetter & Rootzén (1988) for a general discussion.

The idea of declustering data as a means of handling dependence is discussed in some detail by Davison & Smith (1990), though the general idea is considerably older. Estimation of the extremal index is considered by Leadbetter et al. (1989) and also by Smith & Weissman (1994). A scheme for choosing simultaneously the threshold and cluster separation size in an analysis of stationary extremes is proposed by Walshaw (1994). Explicit use of the extremal index for modeling sea-levels is developed by Tawn & Vassie (1989, 1990). A more recent study of the problem of estimating the extremal index of processes that can be observed at different frequencies – say, hourly or daily – is given by Robinson & Tawn (2000).

6
Extremes of Non-stationary Sequences

6.1 Model Structures

Non-stationary processes have characteristics that change systematically thorough time. In the context of environmental processes, non-stationarity is often apparent because of seasonal effects, perhaps due to different climate patterns in different months, or in the form of trends, possibly due to long-term climate changes. Like the presence of temporal dependence, such departures from the simple assumptions that were made in the derivation of the extreme value characterizations in Chapters 3 and 4 challenge the utility of the standard models. In Chapter 5 we were able to demonstrate that, in a certain sense and subject to specified limitations, the usual extreme value limit models are still applicable in the presence of temporal dependence. No such general theory can be established for non-stationary processes. Results are available for some very specialized forms of non-stationarity, but these are generally too restrictive to be of use for describing the patterns of non-stationarity found in real processes. Instead, it is usual to adopt a pragmatic approach of using the standard extreme value models as basic templates that can be enhanced by statistical modeling.

As an example, referring back to the Fremantle annual maximum sea-level data discussed in Example 1.3, asymptotic arguments support the use of the GEV distribution for modeling the maximum sea-level in any year, but the apparent trend in the data raises doubts about the suitability of a model which assumes a constant distribution through time. In this particular example, it seems plausible that the basic level of the annual maximum sea-levels has changed linearly over the observation period, but that in other respects, the distribution is unchanged. Using the notation GEV(μ, σ, ξ) to denote the GEV distribution with parameters μ, σ and ξ, it follows that a suitable model for Z_t, the annual maximum sea-level in year t, might be

$$Z_t \sim \text{GEV}(\mu(t), \sigma, \xi),$$

where

$$\mu(t) = \beta_0 + \beta_1 t$$

for parameters β_0 and β_1. In this way, variations through time in the observed process are modeled as a linear trend in the location parameter of the appropriate extreme value model, which in this case is the GEV distribution. The parameter β_1 corresponds to the annual rate of change in annual maximum sea-level. The time-homogeneous model, which seems more plausible for the annual maximum sea-levels at Port Pirie (see Example 1.1), forms a special case of the time-dependent model, with $\beta_1 = 0$, in which case $\mu = \beta_0$.

More complex changes in μ may also be appropriate. For example, a quadratic model,

$$\mu(t) = \beta_0 + \beta_1 t + \beta_2 t^2,$$

or a change-point model,

$$\mu(t) = \begin{cases} \mu_1 & \text{for } t \leq t_0, \\ \mu_2 & \text{for } t > t_0. \end{cases}$$

Non-stationarity may also be expressed in terms of the other extreme value parameters. For example,

$$\sigma(t) = \exp(\beta_0 + \beta_1 t),$$

where the exponential function is used to ensure that the positivity of σ is respected for all values of t. Extreme value model shape parameters are difficult to estimate with precision, so it is usually unrealistic to try modeling ξ as a smooth function of time. An alternative, that is especially useful for modeling seasonal changes in threshold exceedance models, is to specify a model with different parameters in each season. With a time series of, say, daily observations $X_1, X_2, \ldots$, we denote by $s(t)$ the season into which day t falls. Different thresholds $u_{s(t)}$ might also be appropriate in each of the seasons. Using the notation GP(σ, ξ) to denote the generalized Pareto distribution with parameters σ and ξ, the seasonal model can be expressed as

$$(X_t - u_{s(t)} \mid X_t > u_{s(t)}) \sim \text{GP}(\sigma_{s(t)}, \xi_{s(t)}), \tag{6.1}$$

where $(\sigma_{s(t)}, \xi_{s(t)})$ are the generalized Pareto distribution parameters in season $s(t)$. This type of model may be appropriate for the Wooster temperature data of Example 1.7, though the determination of an appropriate segregation into seasons is itself an issue.

A different situation which may arise is that the extremal behavior of one series is related to that of another variable, referred to as a **covariate**. For example, in an extreme value analysis of pollution concentrations, the extent of a high pollutant level may be dependent on the concurrent wind speed (strong winds having a dispersive effect). Figure 1.4 suggested a similar phenomenon for annual maximum sea-levels at Fremantle, which appear greater in years for which the mean value of the Southern Oscillation Index is higher. This suggests the following model for Z_t, the annual maximum sea-level in year t:

$$Z_t \sim \text{GEV}(\mu(t), \sigma, \xi),$$

where

$$\mu(t) = \beta_0 + \beta_1 \text{SOI}(t),$$

and $\text{SOI}(t)$ denotes the Southern Oscillation Index in year t.

There is a unity of structure in all of these examples. In each case the extreme value parameters can be written in the form

$$\theta(t) = h(X^T \beta), \qquad (6.2)$$

where θ denotes either μ, σ or ξ, h is a specified function, β is a vector of parameters, and X is a model vector. In this context, h is usually referred to as the inverse-link function. Returning to the earlier examples, for the linear trend in μ, h is the identity function and

$$\mu(t) = [1, t] \begin{bmatrix} \beta_0 \\ \beta_1 \end{bmatrix}. \qquad (6.3)$$

This expands to

$$\mu(t) = [1, t, t^2] \begin{bmatrix} \beta_0 \\ \beta_1 \\ \beta_2 \end{bmatrix}$$

for the quadratic trend model. The log-linear model for σ has a similar structure to (6.3), with $\sigma(t)$ replacing $\mu(t)$ and with the inverse-link h taken as the exponential function. The seasonal model with k seasons $s_1, \ldots, s_k$ takes the form

$$\mu(t) = [I_1(t), I_2(t), \ldots, I_k(t)] \begin{bmatrix} \beta_1 \\ \beta_2 \\ \vdots \\ \beta_k \end{bmatrix},$$

where $I_j(t)$ is the indicator function

$$I_j(t) = \begin{cases} 1, & \text{if } s(t) = s_j, \\ 0, & \text{otherwise}, \end{cases}$$

and with similar expressions for $\sigma(t)$ and $\xi(t)$. Finally, the SOI covariate model may be expressed as

$$\mu(t) = [1, \text{SOI}(t)] \begin{bmatrix} \beta_0 \\ \beta_1 \end{bmatrix}. \tag{6.4}$$

There is a similarity between the class of models implied by (6.2) and generalized linear models (GLMs), whose theory is well developed and for which estimating algorithms are routinely provided in statistical software. The analogy is not close enough, however, for any of the standard results or computational tools to be directly transferable to the extreme value context. The main difference is that the GLM family is restricted to distributions that are within the exponential family of distributions; the standard extreme value models generally fall outside of this family. Nonetheless, (6.2) applied to any or each of the parameters in an extreme value model provides a broad and attractive family for representing non-stationarity in extreme value datasets.

6.2 Inference

6.2.1 Parameter Estimation

An advantage of maximum likelihood over other techniques of parameter estimation is its adaptability to changes in model structure. Take, for example, a non-stationary GEV model to describe the distribution of Z_t for $t = 1, \ldots, m$:

$$Z_t \sim \text{GEV}(\mu(t), \sigma(t), \xi(t)),$$

where each of $\mu(t), \sigma(t)$ and $\xi(t)$ have an expression in terms of a parameter vector and covariates of the type (6.2). Denoting by β the complete vector of parameters, the likelihood is simply

$$L(\beta) = \prod_{t=1}^{m} g(z_t; \mu(t), \sigma(t), \xi(t)),$$

where $g(z_t; \mu(t), \sigma(t), \xi(t))$ denotes the GEV density function with parameters $\mu(t), \sigma(t), \xi(t)$ evaluated at z_t. Hence, by analogy with (3.7), if none of the $\xi(t)$ is zero, the log-likelihood is

$$\ell(\mu, \sigma, \xi) = -\sum_{t=1}^{m} \left\{ \log \sigma(t) + (1 + 1/\xi(t)) \log \left[1 + \xi(t) \left(\frac{z_t - \mu(t)}{\sigma(t)} \right) \right] \right. \\ \left. + \left[1 + \xi(t) \left(\frac{z_t - \mu(t)}{\sigma(t)} \right) \right]^{-1/\xi(t)} \right\}, \tag{6.5}$$

provided that

$$1 + \xi(t)\left(\frac{z_t - \mu(t)}{\sigma(t)}\right) > 0, \text{ for } t = 1,\ldots,m,$$

where $\mu(t), \sigma(t)$ and $\xi(t)$ are replaced by their expressions in terms of β according to the chosen model structure determined by (6.2). If any of the $\xi(t) = 0$, it is necessary to use the appropriate limiting form as $\xi(t) \to 0$ in (6.5), as in the replacement of the GEV likelihood (3.7) by the Gumbel likelihood (3.9). Numerical techniques can be used to maximize (6.5), yielding the maximum likelihood estimate of β. Approximate standard errors and confidence intervals follow in the usual way from the observed information matrix, which can also be evaluated numerically.

6.2.2 Model Choice

With the possibility of modeling any combination of the extreme value model parameters as functions of time or other covariates, there is a large catalogue of models to choose from, and selecting an appropriate model becomes an important issue. The basic principle is parsimony, obtaining the simplest model possible, that explains as much of the variation in the data as possible. For example, when modeling the annual maximum sea-level data of Example 1.3, it looks certain that a linear trend component will be needed, probably in the location parameter μ. But perhaps a quadratic trend is also evident? Since the class of quadratic models includes the linear models as a special case, such a model is bound to improve on the linear model in terms of the accuracy in describing variations in the observed data. However, the model is required as a description of the process that generated the data, not for the data themselves, so it is necessary to assess the strength of evidence for the more complex model structure. If the evidence is not particularly strong, the simpler model should be chosen in preference.

As discussed in Section 2.6.6, maximum likelihood estimation of nested models leads to a simple test procedure of one model against the other. With models $\mathcal{M}_0 \subset \mathcal{M}_1$, the deviance statistic is defined as

$$D = 2\{\ell_1(\mathcal{M}_1) - \ell_0(\mathcal{M}_0)\},$$

where $\ell_0(\mathcal{M}_0)$ and $\ell_1(\mathcal{M}_1)$ are the maximized log-likelihoods under models $\mathcal{M}_0$ and $\mathcal{M}_1$ respectively. Large values of D indicate that model $\mathcal{M}_1$ explains substantially more of the variation in the data than $\mathcal{M}_0$; small values of D suggest that the increase in model size does not bring worthwhile improvements in the model's capacity to explain the data. Help in determining how large D should be before model $\mathcal{M}_1$ is preferred to model $\mathcal{M}_0$ is provided by the asymptotic distribution of the deviance function. This is summarized in Theorem 2.7, which states that model $\mathcal{M}_0$ is rejected by a test at the α-level of significance if $D > c_\alpha$, where c_α is the $(1-\alpha)$ quantile of the χ_k^2 distribution, and k is the difference in the dimensionality of $\mathcal{M}_1$ and $\mathcal{M}_0$. In other words, a formal criterion can be given to specify how large D should be before model $\mathcal{M}_1$ is to be preferred. There is still subjectivity in the choice of α, whose value determines the compromise between the two types of error that can be made – wrongly adopting $\mathcal{M}_1$, or wrongly sticking with $\mathcal{M}_0$ – but this balancing act is unavoidable. For non-nested models, a variety of modifications to the deviance-based criterion have been proposed (Cox & Hinkley, 1974, for example).

6.2.3 Model Diagnostics

Having estimated a range of possible models and selected between them, we need to ensure that the final model adopted is actually a good representation of the data. We discussed in Chapters 3 and 4 procedures for model-checking when data are assumed to be identically distributed, but in the non-stationary case the lack of homogeneity in the distributional assumptions for each observation means some modification is needed. It is generally only possible to apply such diagnostic checks to a standardized version of the data, conditional on the fitted parameter values.[1] For example, on the basis of an estimated model

$$Z_t \sim \text{GEV}(\hat{\mu}(t), \hat{\sigma}(t), \hat{\xi}(t)),$$

the standardized variables $\tilde{Z}_t$, defined by

$$\tilde{Z}_t = \frac{1}{\hat{\xi}(t)} \log\left\{1 + \hat{\xi}(t)\left(\frac{Z_t - \hat{\mu}(t)}{\hat{\sigma}(t)}\right)\right\}, \tag{6.6}$$

each have the standard Gumbel distribution, with probability distribution function

$$\Pr\{\tilde{Z}_t \leq z\} = \exp\{-e^{-z}\}, \quad z \in \mathbb{R}. \tag{6.7}$$

This means that probability and quantile plots of the observed $\tilde{z}_t$ can be made with reference to distribution (6.7). Denoting the ordered values of the $\tilde{z}_t$ by $\tilde{z}_{(1)}, \ldots, \tilde{z}_{(m)}$, the probability plot consists of the pairs

$$\{i/(m+1), \exp(-\exp(-\tilde{z}_{(i)})); \; i = 1, \ldots, m\},$$

while the quantile plot is comprised of the pairs

$$\left\{\left(\tilde{z}_{(i)}, -\log\left(-\log(i/(m+1))\right)\right); \; i = 1, \ldots, m\right\}.$$

The probability plot is invariant to the choice of Gumbel as a reference distribution, but the quantile plot is not: choices other than Gumbel would

---

[1] A similar procedure was adopted for the example in Section 2.7.

lead to a different plot. Notwithstanding this arbitrariness, the choice of Gumbel is arguably the most natural given its status within the GEV family.

Similar techniques can be adopted for the generalized Pareto distribution. In this case, we have a set of thresholds $u(t)$ that are possibly time-varying, leading to threshold excesses $y_{t_1}, \ldots y_{t_k}$.[2] The estimated model, in its general form, is

$$Y_t \sim \text{GP}(\hat{\sigma}(t), \hat{\xi}(t)).$$

This time, since the exponential distribution is a special case of the generalized Pareto family with $\xi \to 0$, it is more natural to apply a transformation to a standard exponential distribution:

$$\tilde{Y}_{t_k} = \frac{1}{\hat{\xi}(t)} \log \left\{ 1 + \hat{\xi}(t) \left(\frac{Y_{t_k} - u_t}{\hat{\sigma}(t)} \right) \right\}.$$

Denoting the ordered values of the observed $\tilde{Y}_{t_j}$ by $\tilde{y}_{(1)}, \ldots, \tilde{y}_{(k)}$, it follows that a probability plot can be formed by the pairs

$$\left\{ (i/(k+1), 1 - \exp(-\tilde{y}_{(i)})) \, ; \, i = 1, \ldots, k \right\},$$

and a quantile plot by the pairs

$$\left\{ (\tilde{y}_{(i)}, -\log(1 - i/(k+1))) \, ; \, i = 1, \ldots, k \right\}.$$

As with the GEV distribution, the probability plot is invariant to the choice of reference distribution, but the quantile plot is specific to the choice of exponential scale.

6.3 Examples

6.3.1 Annual Maximum Sea-levels

Returning to the discussion of Examples 1.1 and 1.3, there appeared to be visual evidence of a trend in the Fremantle series, but not in the Port Pirie series. The strength of evidence for these conclusions can now be assessed through modeling, which also leads to estimates of the magnitude of any apparent trends.

We obtained in Section 3.4.1 that the maximized log-likelihood for the stationary $\text{GEV}(\mu, \sigma, \xi)$ model fitted to the Port Pirie data is 4.34. Allowing a linear trend in μ has a maximized log-likelihood of 4.37. Consequently, the deviance statistic for comparing these two models is $D = 2(4.37 - 4.34) = 0.06$. This value is small on the scale of a χ_1^2 distribution, implying there is no evidence of a linear trend, and confirming the view reached by visual inspection of the data.

---

[2] The notation y_{t_j} is used here to emphasize the fact that the jth threshold excess is unlikely to correspond to the jth observation in the original process.

112   6. Extremes of Non-stationary Sequences

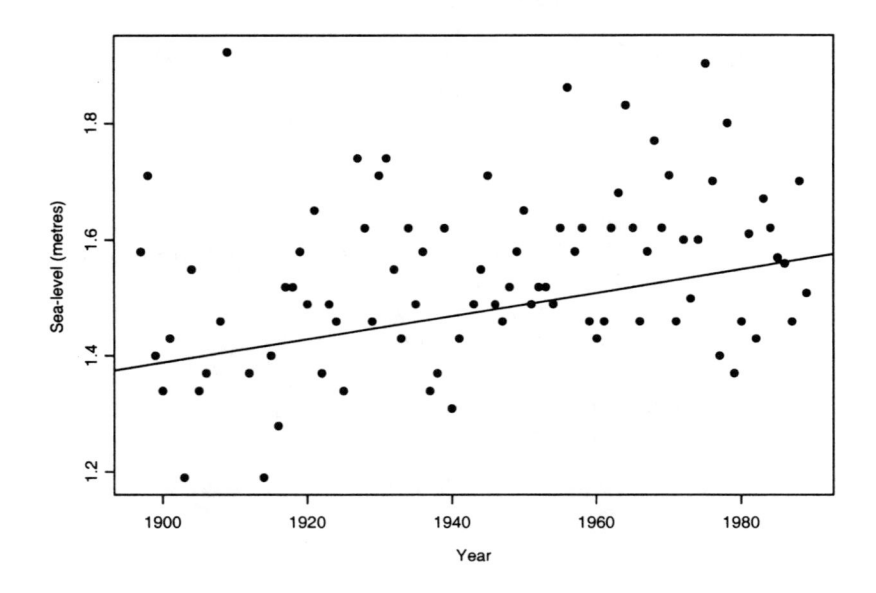

FIGURE 6.1. Fitted estimates for μ in linear trend GEV model of Fremantle annual maximum sea-level series.

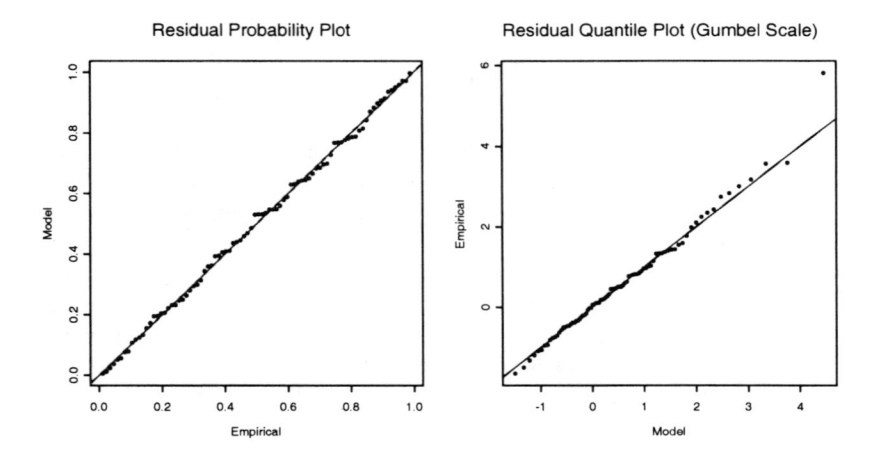

FIGURE 6.2. Residual diagnostic plots in linear trend GEV model of Fremantle annual maximum sea-level series.

It is a different story for the Fremantle data. The stationary GEV model for these data leads to a maximized log-likelihood of 43.6. Allowing a linear trend in μ has a maximized log-likelihood of 49.9. The deviance statistic for comparing these two models is therefore $D = 2(49.4 - 43.6) = 11.6$. This value is overwhelmingly large when compared to a χ_1^2 distribution, implying that the linear trend component explains a substantial amount of the variation in the data, and is likely to be a genuine effect in the sea-level process rather than a chance feature in the observed data. Writing $\mu(t) = \beta_0 + \beta_1 t$, where t is an index for year, with $t = 1$ corresponding to 1897,[3] the maximum likelihood estimate is $\hat{\beta}_0 = 1.38$ (0.03), $\hat{\beta}_1 = 0.00203$ (0.00052), $\hat{\sigma} = 0.124$ (0.010) and $\hat{\xi} = -0.125$ (0.070), with standard errors in parentheses. Therefore, the estimated rise in annual maximum sea-levels is around 2 mm per year, and although this value is not particularly large, the evidence supporting such an effect is strong. There is no evidence supporting either a quadratic trend in μ or a linear trend in σ: the maximized log-likelihoods for the corresponding models are 50.6 and 50.7 respectively, so that tests based on the associated deviance statistics imply no significant improvement over the linear model in μ. The linear trend in μ is plotted relative to the original series in Fig. 6.1. The quality of the fitted model is supported by diagnostic plots applied to residuals, as described in Section 6.2.3. For the Fremantle data, these plots are shown in Fig. 6.2.

We also discussed in Chapter 1 the apparent tendency for annual maximum sea-levels at Fremantle to be greater in years for which the mean value of the Southern Oscillation Index (SOI) is high. This is of particular interest, since the SOI is often used as a proxy for abnormal meteorological activity on a global scale, such as the El Niño effect. Establishing a relationship between extreme sea-levels and SOI is therefore useful in understanding the dynamics that determine abnormal sea-states. Fitting the model in which the GEV location parameter is linearly related to SOI – model (6.4) – leads to a maximized log-likelihood of 47.2. Compared with the stationary model log-likelihood of 43.6, we obtain a deviance statistic that is large on the scale of a χ_1^2 distribution, suggesting the presence of a relationship. But the full picture is more complicated. We have already established a linear trend in μ, so it is possible that SOI is also time-varying, and that the apparent association between extreme sea-levels and SOI is simply a consequence of their mutual change over time. To consider this possibility, it is necessary to expand model (6.4) to

$$\mu(t) = [1, t, \mathrm{SOI}(t)] \begin{bmatrix} \beta_0 \\ \beta_1 \\ \beta_2 \end{bmatrix},$$

---

[3]There are a number of years with missing data, so t runs from 1 to 93, though there are just 86 observations.

114   6. Extremes of Non-stationary Sequences

TABLE 6.1. Maximized log-likelihoods and parameter estimates, with standard errors in parentheses, of various models for $\tilde{\mu}$ in GEV model for minima applied to race time data of Example 1.4

Model	Log-likelihood	$\hat{\beta}$	$\hat{\sigma}$	$\hat{\xi}$
Constant	-54.5	239.3	3.63	-0.469
		(0.9)	(0.64)	(0.141)
Linear	-51.8	$(242.9, -0.311)$	2.72	-0.201
		(1.4, 0.101)	(0.49)	(0.172)
Quadratic	-48.4	$(247.0, -1.395, 0.049)$	2.28	-0.182
		(2.3, 0.420, 0.018)	(0.45)	(0.232)

so that μ is modeled as a linear combination of both time and SOI. The maximized log-likelihood of this model is 53.9, so the deviance statistic for comparison with the linear-trend only model is $D = 2(53.9 - 49.9) = 8.0$. Once again, this is large when judged relative to a χ_1^2 distribution, providing evidence that the effect of SOI *is* influential on annual maximum sea-levels at Fremantle, even after the allowance for time-variation. The estimated value of β_2 in this model is 0.055, with a standard error of 0.020, so that every unit increase in SOI results in an estimated increase of around 5.5 cm in annual maximum sea-level. The estimated time trend in this model remains unchanged at around 2 mm per year.

6.3.2   Race Time Data

Even a casual look at Fig. 1.5 suggests that the race times in Example 1.4 have improved considerably over the observation period. This conclusion can be confirmed and quantified by a likelihood analysis. Using the notation $\text{GEV}_m(\mu, \sigma, \xi)$ to denote the GEV distribution for minima, we model the race time Z_t in year indexed by t as

$$Z_t \sim \text{GEV}_m(\tilde{\mu}(t), \sigma(t), \xi(t)).$$

Equivalently, by the argument in Chapter 3,

$$-Z_t \sim \text{GEV}(\mu(t), \sigma(t), \xi(t)),$$

with $\tilde{\mu}(t) = -\mu(t)$. The motivation for this model is that fastest race times in each year are the minima of many such race times. But because of overall improvements in athletic performance, the distribution is non-homogeneous across years. Fig. 1.5 suggests that the change in distribution through time affects the level of the distribution, rather than other aspects, leading again to a model in which $\sigma(t)$ and $\xi(t)$ are assumed constant, but $\tilde{\mu}(t)$ is modeled.

A summary of results for the models with constant, linear and quadratic trends in $\tilde{\mu}(t)$ is given in Table 6.1. From the log-likelihoods, deviance

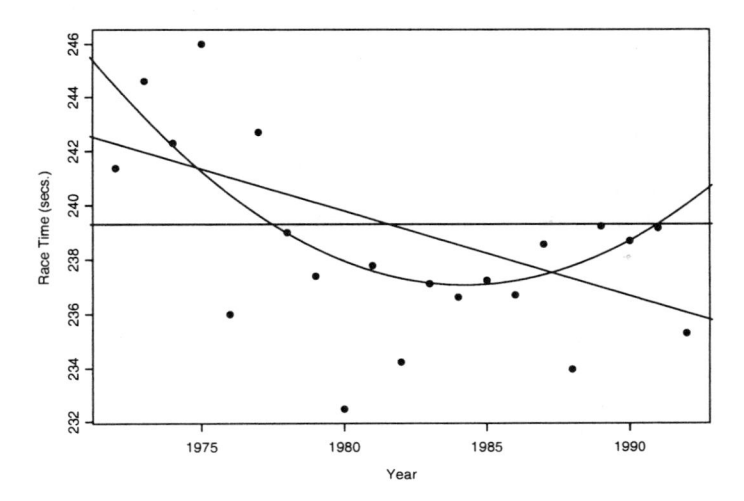

FIGURE 6.3. Fitted estimates for $\tilde{\mu}$ in GEV model for minima applied to fastest annual race times for women's 1500 meters event.

statistics to compare the linear and constant models, and the quadratic and linear models, are 5.4 and 6.8 respectively. Since both values are large when compared to a χ_1^2 distribution, it follows that the linear model improves on the constant model, but that the quadratic model does better still. Looking at the sign of the parameter estimates in the quadratic model, the linear component is negative, while the quadratic term is positive. This implies a decelerated annual improvement in race times. Using a cubic model results in a negligible change in maximized log-likelihood with respect to the quadratic model; the higher-order model can therefore be discarded.

Table 6.1 illustrates another reason why it is important to model nonstationarity as carefully as possible. The estimated shape parameter in the homogeneous-$\tilde{\mu}$ model is -0.469. The corresponding estimate in the better-fitting quadratic model is -0.182. Though the difference is not so great once sampling error is accounted for, the point is that model misspecification of one parameter can lead to distorted estimates of another. That is, if any part of the variation in data is due to systematic effects, such as time variation, that are not modeled or are mis-modeled, substantial bias can arise in the estimation of the random part of the model. In the case of extreme value analyses, since the models are likely to be used for extrapolation, serious and expensive errors may result.

Fig. 6.3 shows the estimated trend for $\tilde{\mu}$ using the constant, linear and quadratic models. As suggested by the likelihood analysis, the quadratic model gives the most faithful representation of the apparent time variation in the data, but the quadratic coefficient leads to an increase in $\tilde{\mu}(t)$, and hence in the level of fastest race times, from around 1984 onwards. This reflects the apparent slowing-down in the reduction of race times. However, from general knowledge about the context of the data, it is difficult to believe that the level of fastest race times has actually worsened in recent years. It is much more likely that this conclusion is an artifact of working with a quadratic model that is bound to imply an increase in $\tilde{\mu}(t)$ at some point, even if not within the range of the observed data. This difficulty can be avoided by imposing a model structure on $\tilde{\mu}(t)$ that is monotonic in t; for example,

$$\tilde{\mu}(t) = \beta_0 + \beta_1 e^{-\beta_2 t}. \tag{6.8}$$

Though it is not difficult to write a purpose-built routine to fit such a model by maximum likelihood, it falls outside of the class of models implied by (6.2), and is therefore not immediately fitted using the software described in the Appendix. However, if β_0 is fixed,

$$Z_t - \beta_0 \sim \text{GEV}_m(\tilde{\mu}(t), \sigma, \xi), \tag{6.9}$$

where

$$\tilde{\mu}(t) = \beta_1 e^{-\beta_2 t},$$

which can be rewritten as

$$\tilde{\mu}(t) = h(\tilde{\beta}_1 + \tilde{\beta}_2 t),$$

where $h(x) = \exp(x)$, $\tilde{\beta}_1 = \log(\beta_1)$ and $\tilde{\beta}_2 = -\beta_2$. So, with β_0 known, model (6.8) does fall within the class defined by (6.2). This enables an iterative method of estimation: for a range of values of β_0, the likelihood of model (6.9) is maximized using standard routines. Choosing the maximum of these maximized likelihoods yields the maximum likelihood estimator of β in model (6.8).

Applying this procedure to the race time data leads to the maximum likelihood estimate of $\beta = (237.5, -10.7, 0.223)$, and a maximized log-likelihood of -49.5. The corresponding estimated curve $\tilde{\mu}(t)$ is shown in Fig. 6.4. It is arguable whether the exponential model provides a better description of the data than the quadratic model plotted in Fig. 6.3, but it now respects the constraint that the basic level of fastest race times should be monotonic. Formal comparison between the models is not possible using the deviance statistic, as the models are non-nested. Informally, since the number of parameters in each of the models is equal, the marginally greater log-likelihood of the quadratic model gives it a slight preference. However, the difference in log-likelihoods is slight, and definitely not large enough to lead to rejection of the exponential model if the monotonicity is thought to be a desirable feature.

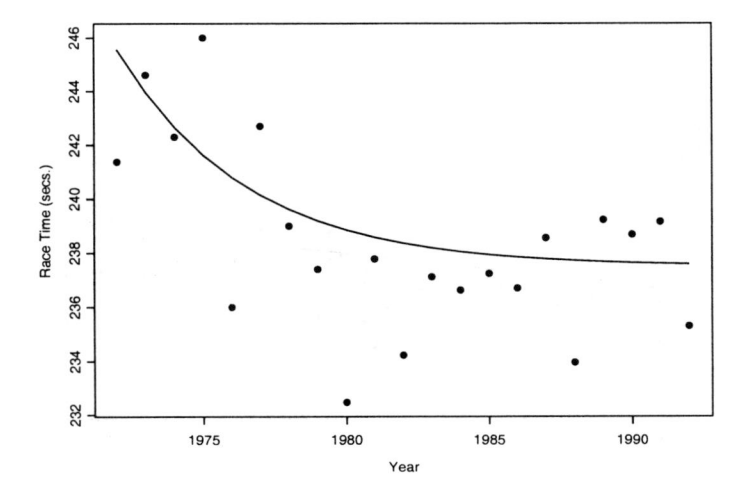

FIGURE 6.4. Fitted estimates for exponential $\tilde{\mu}$ in GEV model for minima applied to fastest annual race times for women's 1500 meters event.

TABLE 6.2. Maximized log-likelihoods, parameter estimates and standard errors (in parentheses) of r largest order statistic model fitted to Venice sea-level data with different values of r. The model is parameterized as $\mu(t) = \beta_0 + \beta_1 t$, where t is a year index running from 1 to 51.

r	Log-lik.	β_0	β_1	σ	ξ
1	−216.1	97.0 (4.2)	0.56 (0.14)	14.6 (1.6)	−0.027 (0.083)
5	−704.8	104.2 (2.0)	0.46 (0.06)	12.3 (0.8)	−0.037 (0.042)
10	−1093.9	104.3 (1.6)	0.48 (0.04)	11.6 (0.6)	−0.070 (0.026)

6.3.3 Venice Sea-level Data

The analysis of the Venice sea-level data using the r largest order statistic model of Section 3.5.3 led to unsatisfactory fits for all choices of r. The plot of the data in Fig. 1.6 suggests why: there is strong visual evidence for a trend. Consequently, the basic r largest order statistic model is distorted, as a substantial part of the variability in the data should properly be explained by the systematic time variation. This again suggests a model in which the location parameter, now in the r largest order statistic model, is linear in time.

Table 6.2 gives values of the maximized log-likelihood, parameter estimates and standard errors for this model using $r = 1, 5$ and 10. These fits are analogous to those summarized in Table 3.1, but with the inclusion of

118   6. Extremes of Non-stationary Sequences

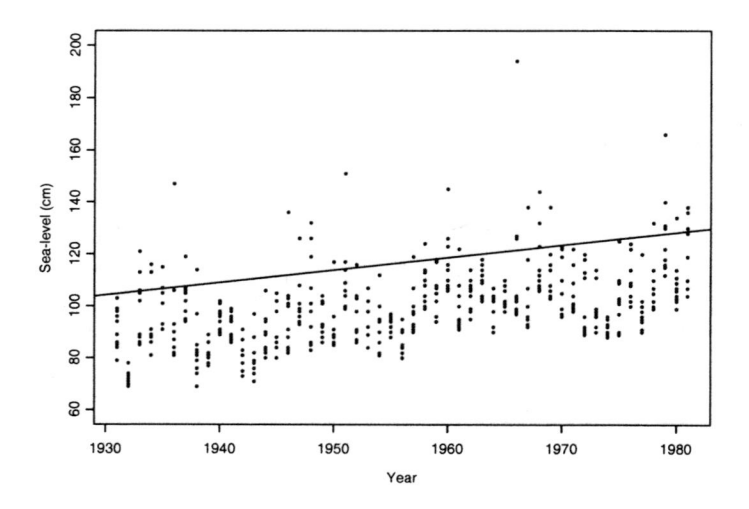

FIGURE 6.5. Estimated linear trend for μ in r largest order statistic model applied to Venice sea-levels with $r = 10$.

the trend parameter. There are several points to be made. First, comparing the log-likelihoods in the two tables, it is clear that for any choice of r, the evidence for a trend of around 0.5 cm per year is overwhelming. Next, there is much greater stability in the parameter estimates across different choices of r in Table 6.2, compared with Table 3.1. Consequently, once the non-stationarity is allowed for in the form of a trend in location, the asymptotic arguments in support of the r largest order statistic model have a much stronger empirical basis. In fact, on the evidence from Table 6.2, the estimates obtained using $r = 10$ are consistent with those of $r = 1$, but with substantially smaller standard errors. It therefore seems reasonable to adopt the $r = 10$ model. The corresponding estimated trend function for μ is superimposed on the data in Fig. 6.5.

As with the non-stationary GEV model, model validity can be checked by producing probability and quantile plots of standardized fitted values. In this case, applying transformation (6.6) leads to a sample of vectors which, under the validity of the fitted model, is such that each vector of order statistics constitutes an independent realization from the r largest order statistic model, with $\mu = 0, \sigma = 1$ and $\xi = 0$. Applying this procedure to the Venice sea-level data, on the basis of the $r = 5$ model, leads to the plots shown in Fig. 6.6. Compared with the corresponding plots in Fig. 3.10, the quality of fit is much improved. Remaining lack-of-fit is likely to be explained, at least in part, by the fact that the apparent cyclicity in the Venice series has not been modeled.

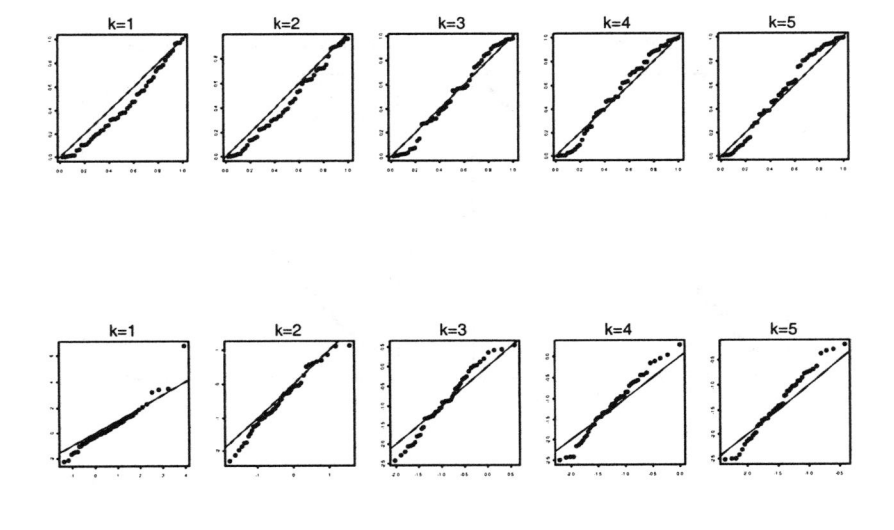

FIGURE 6.6. Model diagnostics for the Venice sea-level data based on the fitted r largest order statistic model with $r = 5$ and trend in location parameter. Plots shown are probability and quantile plots for kth largest order statistic, $k = 1, \ldots, 5$.

6.3.4 Daily Rainfall Data

For the daily rainfall data of Example 1.6, fitting the generalized Pareto distribution with a linear trend in the log-scale parameter,

$$\sigma(t) = \exp(\beta_0 + \beta_1 t),$$

leads to a maximized log-likelihood of -484.6. This compares with the value of -485.1 obtained previously under the time-homogeneous model. The similarity of these values implies there is no evidence of a time trend. For reference, the probability and quantile plots of the transformed residuals of the time-trend model are shown in Fig. 6.7.

6.3.5 Wooster Temperature Data

For the Wooster temperature series discussed in Example 1.7, we observed a strong non-stationarity in the series within each year. Fig. 6.8 shows the data stratified by season. Evidence of non-stationarity remains within each season's data, but to a lesser extent than in the original series. A more

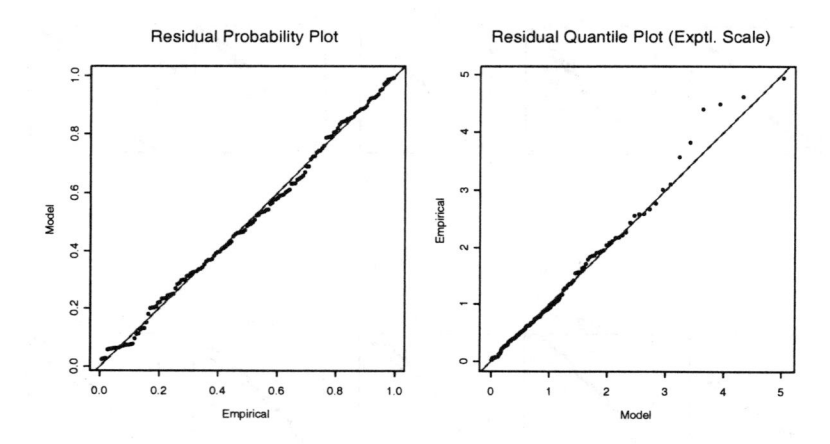

FIGURE 6.7. Probability and quantile plots for residuals in linear trend threshold excess model fitted to daily rainfall data.

thorough analysis might consider the appropriateness of breaking the series into shorter seasons, perhaps monthly. Since the example is illustrative, we retain the four-season model and also disregard the problem of clustering, though in principle we could apply the techniques of Chapter 5 to decluster each season's data before analysis.

One possible model for these data is the simple seasonal model (6.1). Because the likelihood factorizes across the seasons, it is simpler to treat each season separately, and to sum the four individual log-likelihoods. Working with thresholds of $-10, -25, -50$ and -30, for the winter, spring, autumn and summer seasons respectively, yields a maximized log-likelihood of -645.83.

Standard likelihood techniques also enable an assessment of whether any aspects of the process are homogeneous across seasons. For example, it is plausible that, although the location and scale of the data change across seasons, the tail characteristics are similar. This can be modeled by allowing different scale parameters, but a common shape parameter, for each season, generating a five-parameter model, in place of the original eight parameters. The likelihood no longer factorizes across seasons because of the common value of ξ, but the five-parameter log-likelihood is still easily maximized, yielding a value of -646.08. Consequently, the deviance test statistic for comparing the two models is $2(646.08 - 645.83) = 0.5$, which is small when

6.3 Examples   121

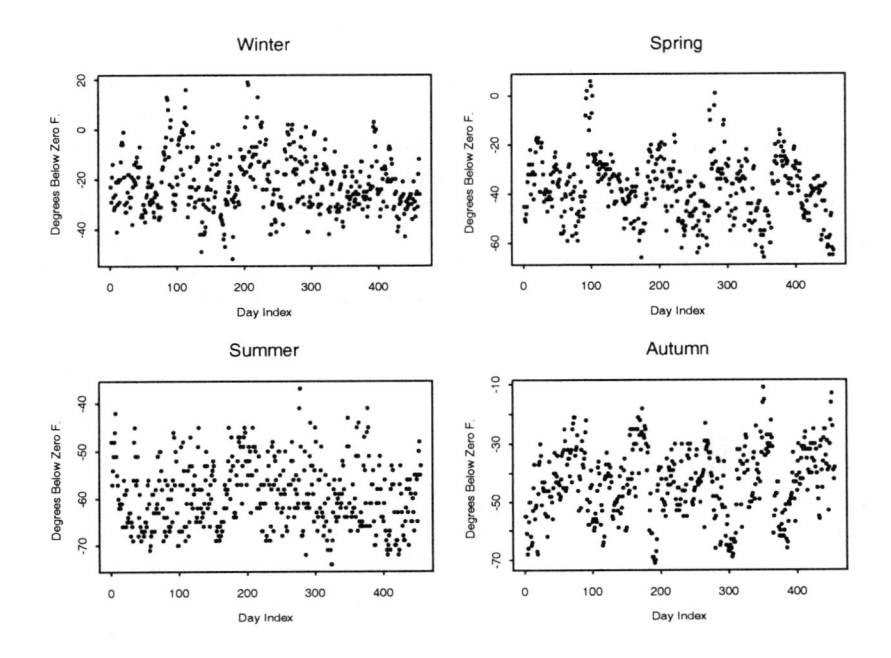

FIGURE 6.8. Negated Wooster temperature series in each of four seasons.

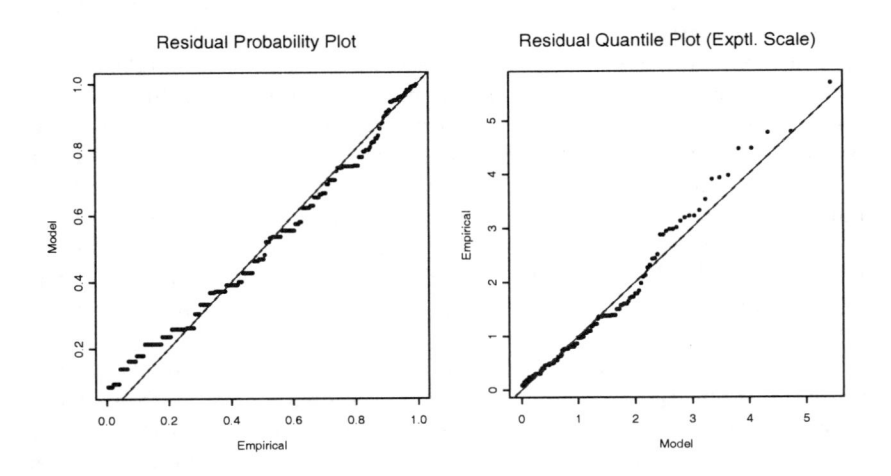

FIGURE 6.9. Diagnostic plots of seasonal-varying scale model for negated Wooster temperature series.

compared to a χ_3^2 distribution. It follows that the constant-ξ model provides an adequate description of the process. The corresponding estimate of ξ is -0.251, with a standard error of 0.059, implying strong evidence for an unbounded tail in each season. It makes little sense to extend this modeling approach to the scale parameter, because of the dependence of the scale parameter on threshold choice (cf. Chapter 4).

Fig. 6.9 gives the transformed probability and quantile plots for the constant-ξ model. The linearity of the plots is reasonable, but not perfect, especially at the lower end of the distribution. This is possibly due to the residual non-stationarity after the seasonal blocking. In Chapter 7 we will discuss a more flexible modeling approach.

6.4 Further Reading

Some simple studies of the theoretical properties of particular classes of non-stationary processes are described by Leadbetter et al. (1983). A number of general results can be found in Hüsler (1986), which also contains further references. A particular application is given by Hüsler (1984). A study of the regularity properties of maximum likelihood in regression-type problems was made by Smith (1989b), generalizing the earlier work in Smith (1985).

For applications, an early reference to the flexibility of maximum likelihood for covariate modeling is Moore (1987). Covariate modeling in the context of the threshold excess model was discussed by Davison & Smith (1990). An alternative technique for modeling extreme value parameters, that accounts for seasonality, was proposed by Zwiers & Ross (1991).

Specific applications have become abundant in recent years. Spatial models for variations in the UK extreme oceanographic climate were developed by Coles & Tawn (1990). These models were taken considerably further in a sequence of studies, culminating in Dixon & Tawn (1999). Similar techniques are also used by Laycock et al. (1990) for estimating the propensity of pits of different sizes in metals due to corrosion, and by Mole et al. (1995) for assessing the dispersive effect of wind sources on pollutant concentrations. A number of other case studies can also be found in Galambos et al. (1994).

Although trends, or other features of a process, may vary smoothly, there are many applications for which such variations do not have the form of low-order polynomials. It is commonplace in general problems of this type to use nonparametric or semiparametric techniques to smooth data. A number of recent references have explored these techniques in an extreme value context. Davison & Ramesh (2000) and Hall & Tajvidi (2000b) each propose the use of local-likelihood techniques. Rosen & Cohen (1994) suggested penalized likelihood for the location parameter of a Gumbel model, and this idea has since been extended to more general extreme value models by Chavez-Demoulin (1999) and Pauli & Coles (2001).

7
A Point Process Characterization of Extremes

7.1 Introduction

There are different ways of characterizing the extreme value behavior of a process, and a particularly elegant formulation is derived from the theory of point processes. The mathematics required for a formal treatment of this theory is outside the scope of this book, but we can again give a more informal development. This requires just basic ideas from point process theory. In a sense, the point process characterization leads to nothing new in terms of statistical models; all inferences made using the point process methodology could equally be obtained using an appropriate model from earlier chapters. However, there are two good reasons for considering this approach. First, it provides an interpretation of extreme value behavior that unifies all the models introduced so far; second, the model leads directly to a likelihood that enables a more natural formulation of non-stationarity in threshold excesses than was obtained from the generalized Pareto model discussed in Chapters 4 and 6.

7.2 Basic Theory of Point Processes

A point process on a set $\mathcal{A}$ is a stochastic rule for the occurrence and position of point events. In a modeling context, with $\mathcal{A}$ representing a period of time, a point process model might be used to describe the occurrence of thunderstorms or earthquakes, for example. From the model, the probability of a certain number of events (thunderstorms/earthquakes) within a specified period could be calculated; or given the occurrence of one event, the expected waiting time until the next. The set $\mathcal{A}$ can also be multi-dimensional. For example, a two-dimensional point process might be used to describe the position of fractures on a glass plate.

One way of characterizing the statistical properties of a point process is to define a set of non-negative integer-valued random variables, $N(A)$, for each $A \subset \mathcal{A}$, such that $N(A)$ is the number of points in the set A. Specifying in a consistent way the probability distribution of each of the $N(A)$ determines the characteristics of the point process, which we label as N. Summary features of a point process can also be defined. In particular,

$$\Lambda(A) = E\{N(A)\},$$

which gives the expected number points in any subset $A \subset \mathcal{A}$, is defined to be the **intensity measure** of the process. Assuming $A = [a_1, x_1] \times \cdots \times [a_k, x_k] \subset \mathbb{R}^k$, and provided it exists, the derivative function

$$\lambda(x) = \frac{\partial \Lambda(A)}{\partial x_1 \cdots \partial x_k}$$

is the **intensity (density) function** of the process.

The canonical point process is the one-dimensional **homogeneous Poisson process**. With a parameter $\lambda > 0$, this is a process on $\mathcal{A} \subset \mathbb{R}$ satisfying:

1. for all $A = [t_1, t_2] \subset \mathcal{A}$,

$$N(A) \sim \text{Poi}(\lambda(t_2 - t_1));$$

2. for all non-overlapping subsets A and B of $\mathcal{A}$, $N(A)$ and $N(B)$ are independent random variables.

In other words, the number of points in a given interval follows a Poisson distribution, with mean proportional to the interval length, and the number of points occurring in separate intervals are mutually independent. The Poisson process, with parameter λ, can be shown to be the appropriate stochastic model for points that occur randomly in time at a uniform of λ per unit time interval. The corresponding intensity measure is $\Lambda([t_1, t_2]) = \lambda(t_2 - t_1)$, and the intensity density function is $\lambda(t) = \lambda$.

The homogeneous Poisson process can be generalized to a model for points that occur randomly in time, but at a variable rate $\lambda(t)$. This leads to the one-dimensional **non-homogeneous Poisson process**, which has the same property of independent counts on non-overlapping subsets as the homogeneous Poisson process, but the modified property that, for all $A = [t_1, t_2] \subset \mathcal{A}$,

$$N(A) \sim \text{Poi}(\Lambda(A)),$$

where
$$\Lambda(A) = \int_{t_1}^{t_2} \lambda(t)dt.$$

Implicitly, the intensity measure and density functions are $\Lambda(\cdot)$ and $\lambda(\cdot)$ respectively.

The non-homogeneous Poisson process generalizes further to provide a description of randomly occurring points in a subset of k-dimensional space. A point process on $\mathcal{A} \subset \mathbb{R}^k$ is said to be a k-dimensional **non-homogeneous Poisson process**, with intensity density function $\lambda(\cdot)$, if it satisfies the property of independent counts on non-overlapping subsets and, for all $A \subset \mathcal{A}$,
$$N(A) \sim \text{Poi}(\Lambda(A)),$$
where
$$\Lambda(A) = \int_A \lambda(\boldsymbol{x})d\boldsymbol{x}.$$

The intrinsic property of a Poisson process is that the points occur independently of one another. The occurrence of a point at a location $x \in \mathcal{A}$ neither encourages, nor inhibits, the occurrence of other points in a neighborhood of x, or in any other location. Poisson processes are therefore ideal candidate models for random scatter. Variations in the number of points in different sub-regions of a space $\mathcal{A}$ are admitted through a non-constant intensity measure function, but this is a consequence of a greater mean number of points in some regions compared with others, not because the presence or absence of points in one set of locations influences the occurrence or location of other points. This also implies that there are physical phenomena for which the Poisson process is a poor model: processes where there is a natural spacing, such as the location of trees in a forest; or processes that have a natural clustering, such as the occurrence times of rainstorms.

Statistical applications of point process models usually require estimation of the process from a set of observed points $x_1, \ldots, x_n$ in a region or interval $\mathcal{A}$. This involves the choice of a class of point process models, followed by estimation within the specified class. We restrict attention to estimation within the family of non-homogeneous Poisson processes. Furthermore, we assume that the intensity function $\lambda(\cdot)$ is within a family of parametric models $\lambda(\cdot; \theta)$, so the only issue, subject to model validity, is the estimation of the unknown parameter vector θ. This parallels our adoption of parametric models for probability distributions in earlier chapters. Of the various estimation procedures available, maximum likelihood again provides a general methodology with attractive qualities.

As usual, the likelihood is derived by regarding the probability of the observed data configuration as a function of the unknown parameter θ. We give the development in the simplest case, where $\mathcal{A}$ is one-dimensional, but the argument is similar for Poisson processes in higher dimensions.

So, suppose points $x_1, \ldots, x_n$ have been observed in a region $\mathcal{A} \subset \mathbb{R}$, and that these are the realization of a Poisson process on $\mathcal{A}$, with intensity function $\lambda(\cdot; \theta)$, for some value of θ. The information contained in the data is that points have occurred at a number of known locations, but nowhere else in the region. The likelihood is derived using both these pieces of information. We let $I_i = [x_i, x_i + \delta_i]$, for $i = 1, \ldots, n$, be a set of small intervals based around the observations, and write $\mathcal{I} = \mathcal{A} \setminus \bigcup_{i=1}^{n} I_i$. By the Poisson property,

$$\Pr\{N(I_i) = 1\} = \exp\{-\Lambda(I_i; \theta)\} \Lambda(I_i; \theta), \tag{7.1}$$

where

$$\Lambda(I_i; \theta) = \int_{x_i}^{x_i + \delta_i} \lambda(u) du \approx \lambda(x_i) \delta_i. \tag{7.2}$$

Substituting (7.2) in (7.1) gives

$$\Pr\{N(I_i) = 1\} \approx \exp\{-\lambda(x_i)\delta_i\} \lambda(x_i)\delta_i \approx \lambda(x_i)\delta_i,$$

where we have used the fact that $\exp\{-\lambda(x_i)\delta_i\} \approx 1$ for small δ_i. Also,

$$\Pr\{N(\mathcal{I}) = 0\} = \exp\{-\Lambda(\mathcal{I})\} \approx \exp\{-\Lambda(\mathcal{A})\},$$

since the δ_i are all small. Hence, the likelihood is

$$\begin{aligned} L(\theta; x_1, \ldots, x_n) &= \Pr\{N(\mathcal{I}) = 0, N(I_1) = 1, N(I_2) = 1, \ldots, N(I_n) = 1\} \\ &= \Pr\{N(\mathcal{I}) = 0\} \prod_{i=1}^{n} \Pr\{N(I_i) = 1\} \\ &\approx \exp\{-\Lambda(\mathcal{A}; \theta)\} \prod_{i=1}^{n} \lambda(x_i; \theta) \delta_i. \end{aligned}$$

Dividing through by the δ_i to obtain a density leads to

$$L(\theta; x_1, \ldots, x_n) = \exp\{-\Lambda(\mathcal{A}; \theta)\} \prod_{i=1}^{n} \lambda(x_i; \theta), \tag{7.3}$$

where

$$\Lambda(\mathcal{A}; \theta) = \int_{\mathcal{A}} \lambda(x; \theta) dx.$$

Likelihood (7.3) is also valid in the more general case of a Poisson process on a k-dimensional set $\mathcal{A}$.

The simplest application of (7.3) is to the situation where $x_1, \ldots, x_n$ are the points of a one-dimensional homogeneous Poisson process, with unknown intensity parameter λ, observed over an interval $\mathcal{A} = [0, t]$. In that case,

$$\Lambda(\mathcal{A}; \lambda) = \lambda t,$$

and so
$$L(\lambda; x_1, \ldots, x_n) = \exp\{-\lambda t\}\lambda^n.$$
As usual, it is easier to maximize the log-likelihood
$$\ell(\lambda) = \log L(\lambda; x_1, \ldots, x_n) = -\lambda t + n \log \lambda,$$
leading to the maximum likelihood estimator
$$\hat{\lambda} = n/t,$$
which is the empirical rate of point occurrence. Maximization of (7.3) for non-homogeneous Poisson process models generally requires numerical techniques.

To exploit point processes as a representation for extreme values, we need a notion of convergence that is the analog of convergence of random variables.

Definition 7.1 Let $N_1, N_2, \ldots$ be a sequence of point processes on $\mathcal{A}$. The sequence is said to **converge in distribution** to N, denoted
$$N_n \xrightarrow{d} N,$$
if, for all choices of m and for all bounded sets $A_1, \ldots, A_m$ such that $\Pr\{N(\partial A_j) = 0\} = 1, j = 1 \ldots, m$, where ∂A is the boundary of A, the joint distribution of $(N_n(A_1), \ldots, N_n(A_m))$ converges in distribution to $(N(A_1), \ldots, N_n(A_m))$. △

Less formally, $N_n \xrightarrow{d} N$ if the probabilistic properties of N_n and N are arbitrarily similar for large enough n.

7.3 A Poisson Process Limit for Extremes

7.3.1 Convergence Law

The point process framework provides an elegant way to formulate extreme value limit results. As in the threshold excess model formulation of Chapter 4, we assume $X_1, X_2, \ldots$ to be a series of independent and identically distributed random variables, with common distribution function F. We suppose that the X_i are well behaved in an extreme value sense. That is, with $M_n = \max\{X_1, \ldots, X_n\}$, that there are sequences of constants $\{a_n > 0\}$ and $\{b_n\}$ such that
$$\Pr\{(M_n - b_n)/a_n \leq z\} \to G(z),$$

with
$$G(z) = \exp\left\{-\left[1 + \xi\left(\frac{z-\mu}{\sigma}\right)\right]^{-1/\xi}\right\}$$

for some parameters $\mu, \sigma > 0$ and ξ. We then define a sequence of point processes N_n on $\mathbb{R}^2$ by

$$N_n = \{(i/(n+1), (X_i - b_n)/a_n) : i = 1, \ldots, n\}.$$

The scaling in the first ordinate ensures that the time axis is always mapped to $(0, 1)$; the scaling in the second ordinate stabilizes the behavior of extremes as $n \to \infty$. The fundamental result, stated more precisely below in Theorem 7.1, is that on regions of the form $[0, 1] \times [u, \infty)$, $N_n \stackrel{d}{\to} N$ as $n \to \infty$, where N is a non-homogeneous Poisson process. An outline of the argument follows.

Consider a region of the form $A = [0, 1] \times (u, \infty)$ for some large value of u. Then, each of the n points of N_n has probability p of falling in A, where

$$p = \Pr\{(X_i - b_n)/a_n > u\} \approx \frac{1}{n}\left[1 + \xi\left(\frac{u-\mu}{\sigma}\right)\right]^{-1/\xi}$$

by (4.7). Since the X_i are mutually independent, $N_n(A)$ has the binomial distribution

$$N_n(A) \sim \text{Bin}(n, p). \tag{7.4}$$

By the standard convergence of a binomial distribution to a Poisson limit, combining (7.4) and (7.2), the limiting distribution of $N_n(A)$ as $n \to \infty$ is $\text{Poi}(\Lambda(A))$, with

$$\Lambda(A) = \left[1 + \xi\left(\frac{u-\mu}{\sigma}\right)\right]^{-1/\xi}.$$

Because of the homogeneity of the process in the time direction, it follows that, for any region of the form $A = [t_1, t_2] \times (u, \infty)$, with $[t_1, t_2] \subset [0, 1]$, the limiting distribution of $N_n(A)$ is also $\text{Poi}(\Lambda(A))$, where

$$\Lambda(A) = (t_2 - t_1)\left[1 + \xi\left(\frac{u-\mu}{\sigma}\right)\right]^{-1/\xi}. \tag{7.5}$$

This Poisson limit for all such sets A, together with the fact that the distributions of the $N(A)$ on non-overlapping sets are bound to be independent by construction, is sufficient to establish the Poisson process limit, with intensity measure of the limiting process given by (7.5). The result is summarized in the following theorem.

Theorem 7.1 Let $X_1, X_2, \ldots$ be a series of independent and identically distributed random variables for which there are sequences of constants $\{a_n > 0\}$ and $\{b_n\}$ such that

$$\Pr\{(M_n - b_n)/a_n \leq z\} \to G(z),$$

where
$$G(z) = \exp\left\{-\left[1+\xi\left(\frac{z-\mu}{\sigma}\right)\right]^{-1/\xi}\right\},$$

and let z_- and z_+ be the lower and upper endpoints of G respectively. Then, the sequence of point processes

$$N_n = \{(i/(n+1), (X_i - b_n)/a_n) : i = 1, \ldots, n\}$$

converges on regions of the form $(0,1) \times [u, \infty)$, for any $u > z_-$, to a Poisson process, with intensity measure on $A = [t_1, t_2] \times [z, z_+)$ given by

$$\Lambda(A) = (t_2 - t_1)\left[1+\xi\left(\frac{z-\mu}{\sigma}\right)\right]^{-1/\xi}. \tag{7.6}$$

□

7.3.2 Examples

We now consider briefly the behavior of the Poisson process limit for the three population models considered previously in Sections 3.1.5 and 4.2.3.

Example 7.1 If $X_1, X_2, \ldots$ is a sequence of independent standard exponential variables, the limit G is the standard Gumbel distribution, with $(z_-, z_+) = (-\infty, \infty)$. Hence,

$$N_n = \{(i/(n+1), (X_i - n)) : i = 1, \ldots, n\}$$

converges to a Poisson process with intensity measure on $A = [t_1, t_2] \times [z, \infty)$, for $z > -\infty$, given by

$$\Lambda(A) = (t_2 - t_1)\exp(-z).$$

This is the limit of (7.6) in the case $\mu = 0$, $\sigma = 1$ as $\xi \to 0$. ▲

Example 7.2 If $X_1, X_2, \ldots$ is a sequence of independent standard Fréchet variables, the limit G is the standard Fréchet distribution, with $(z_-, z_+) = (0, \infty)$. In this case,

$$N_n = \{(i/(n+1), X_i/n) : i = 1, \ldots, n\},$$

and convergence is to a Poisson process with intensity measure on $A = [t_1, t_2] \times [z, \infty)$, for $z > 0$, given by

$$\Lambda(A) = (t_2 - t_1)z^{-1}.$$

This is (7.6), with $\mu = 1$, $\sigma = 1$, $\xi = 1$. ▲

Example 7.3 If $X_1, X_2, \ldots$ is a sequence of independent uniform $U(0,1)$ variables, the limit $G(z) = e^z$, for $z < 0$. Hence, $(z_-, z_+) = (-\infty, 0)$,

$$N_n = \{(i/(n+1), n(X_i - 1)) : i = 1, \ldots, n\},$$

and convergence is to a Poisson process with intensity measure on $A = [t_1, t_2] \times [z, 0]$, for $z < 0$, given by

$$\Lambda(A) = (t_2 - t_1)(-z),$$

which is (7.6), with $\mu = -1$, $\sigma = 1$, $\xi = -1$. ▲

These examples illustrate that the domain of the limiting Poisson process is not related to the endpoints of the distribution of the X_i, but to those of the limit distribution G. In particular, the normalization applied to the points in N_n may be regarded as mapping the non-extreme values close to the lower boundary of $(0,1) \times (z_-, z_+)$. For this reason, the convergence in Theorem 7.1 is valid only on regions that are bounded from z_-.

7.4 Connections with Other Extreme Value Models

It is easy to demonstrate that the block maxima model, the r largest order statistic model and the threshold excess model are all special cases of the point process representation given in Theorem 7.1. There is a circularity in the argument, however, because (4.7) was used in establishing the Poisson limit. Nonetheless, since Theorem 7.1 can also be derived from first principles, the following arguments demonstrate that each of the models of the earlier chapters is consequent on the point process representation.

First, the block maxima result. Denoting $M_n = \max\{X_1, \ldots, X_n\}$ in the usual way, and letting

$$N_n = \{(i/(n+1), (X_i - b_n)/a_n) : i = 1, \ldots, n\},$$

the event $\{(M_n - b_n)/a_n \leq z\}$ is equivalent to the event $N_n(A_z) = 0$, where $A_z = (0,1) \times (z, \infty)$. Hence,

$$\begin{aligned}
\Pr\{(M_n - b_n)/a_n \leq z\} &= \Pr\{N_n(A_z) = 0\} \\
&\rightarrow \Pr\{N(A_z) = 0\} \\
&= \exp\{-\Lambda(A_z)\} \\
&= \exp\left\{-\left[1 + \xi\left(\frac{z-\mu}{\sigma}\right)\right]^{-1/\xi}\right\},
\end{aligned}$$

so the limiting distribution of normalized block maxima is the GEV distribution.

Similar arguments apply for the threshold excess model. First, it is helpful to factorize $\Lambda(A_z)$ as

$$\Lambda(A_z) = \Lambda_1([t_1, t_2]) \times \Lambda_2([z, \infty)),$$

where

$$\Lambda_1([t_1, t_2]) = (t_2 - t_1) \quad \text{and} \quad \Lambda_2([z, \infty)) = \left[1 + \xi\left(\frac{z-\mu}{\sigma}\right)\right]^{-1/\xi}.$$

Then,

$$\begin{aligned}
\Pr\{(X_i - b_n)/a_n > z \mid (X_i - b_n)/a_n > u\} &= \frac{\Lambda_2[z, \infty)}{\Lambda_2[u, \infty)} \\
&= \frac{n^{-1}\left[1 + \xi(z-\mu)/\sigma\right]^{-1/\xi}}{n^{-1}\left[1 + \xi(u-\mu)/\sigma\right]^{-1/\xi}} \\
&= \left[1 + \frac{\xi(z-\mu)/\sigma}{1 + \xi(u-\mu)/\sigma}\right]^{-1/\xi} \\
&= \left[1 + \xi\left(\frac{z-u}{\tilde{\sigma}}\right)\right]^{-1/\xi},
\end{aligned}$$

with $\tilde{\sigma} = \sigma + \xi(u-\mu)$. Absorbing the scaling coefficients a_n and b_n in the usual way leads to (4.7).

Derivation of the r largest order statistic characterization is deferred until Section 7.9.

7.5 Statistical Modeling

Because of the connections between the two approaches, any inference made using the point process characterization of extremes could equally be made using the threshold excess model. There are advantages, however, in working directly with the point process model. As with all of the extreme value models, it is usual to interpret the limiting model – in this case the Poisson process – as a reasonable approximation for large but finite sample behavior. That is, in the point process convergence of $N_n \to N$, to assume that the probability laws associated with the limit N provide a reasonable approximation to those of N_n for large enough n. Since the convergence is restricted to sets that exclude the lower boundary, the approximation is likely to be good only on sets of the form $(0, 1) \times (u, \infty)$, for large enough u. In other words, Theorem 7.1 provides a representation only for extreme value behavior of the X_i, and for practical application, it is necessary to make judgements as to what level of u is extreme enough for the limit to provide a reasonable approximation.

Another issue concerns the normalizing sequences $\{a_n\}$ and $\{b_n\}$. As with the earlier extreme value models, these are dependent on the underlying distribution F of the X_i, and so are unknown in practice. This difficulty is resolved, as in previous models, by absorbing the coefficients into the location and scale parameters of the model.

In summary, Theorem 7.1 can be re-stated in the following form.

Theorem 7.1.1 Let $X_1, \ldots, X_n$ be a series of independent and identically distributed random variables, and let

$$N_n = \{(i/(n+1), X_i) : i = 1, \ldots, n\}.$$

Then, for sufficiently large u, on regions of the form $(0,1) \times [u, \infty)$, N_n is approximately a Poisson process, with intensity measure on $A = [t_1, t_2] \times (z, \infty)$ given by

$$\Lambda(A) = (t_2 - t_1) \left[1 + \xi \left(\frac{z - \mu}{\sigma}\right)\right]^{-1/\xi}. \tag{7.7}$$

□

Theorem 7.1.1 enables the following procedure for modeling extremes within the point process framework. First, select a high threshold u, for which the Poisson approximation is thought to be reasonable, and set $A = (0,1) \times [u, \infty)$.[1] The $N(A)$ points that are observed in the region A are re-labeled $\{(t_1, x_1), \ldots, (t_{N(A)}, x_{N(A)})\}$. Assuming the limiting Poisson process is an acceptable approximation to the process of N_n on A, an approximate likelihood can be derived. Maximizing this likelihood leads to estimates of the parameters (μ, σ, ξ) of the limiting intensity function. A small adjustment is useful at this point: it is conventional to express extreme value limits in terms of approximate distributions of *annual* maxima, rather than, say, 10- or 50-year maxima. Using Theorem 7.1.1 directly means that, if data have been observed for m years, the parameters of the point process likelihood will correspond to the GEV distribution of the m-year maximum. Though an adjustment can always be made post-analysis, it is more straightforward to replace (7.7) with

$$\Lambda(A) = n_y(t_2 - t_1) \left[1 + \xi \left(\frac{z - \mu}{\sigma}\right)\right]^{-1/\xi}, \tag{7.8}$$

where n_y is the number of years of observation. In this case, the estimated parameters (μ, σ, ξ) correspond immediately to the GEV parameters of the annual maximum distribution of the observed process.

---

[1] Choosing a threshold for this model involves the same considerations as for the threshold excess model; see Chapter 4.

Substituting (7.8), with $[t_1, t_2] = [0, 1]$, into the general form of the Poisson process likelihood (7.3) leads to the likelihood function

$$L_A(\mu, \sigma, \xi; x_1, \ldots, x_n) = \exp\{-\Lambda(A)\} \prod_{i=1}^{N(A)} \lambda(t_i, x_i)$$

$$\propto \exp\left\{-n_y \left[1 + \xi\left(\frac{u-\mu}{\sigma}\right)\right]^{-1/\xi}\right\} \prod_{i=1}^{N(A)} \sigma^{-1} \left[1 + \xi\left(\frac{x_i-\mu}{\sigma}\right)\right]^{-\frac{1}{\xi}-1}.$$

(7.9)

This function can be treated in the usual way to obtain maximum likelihood estimates, standard errors and approximate confidence intervals of the model parameters.

Like the threshold excess model, the estimates derived from the point process likelihood are based on all those data that are extreme, in the sense of being greater than a specified threshold. Inferences are therefore likely to be more accurate than estimates based on a direct fit of the GEV distribution to the annual maximum data themselves. As an example, applying this model to the daily rainfall data with a threshold of $u = 30$ yields maximum likelihood estimates $\hat{\mu} = 39.55$ (1.20), $\hat{\sigma} = 9.20$ (0.93) and $\hat{\xi} = 0.184$ (0.101), with standard errors given in parentheses. Because of the parameterization of the model, these parameters are the estimates of GEV parameters for the corresponding annual maximum distribution. Referring back to the threshold excess model analysis of these data in Section 4.4.1 confirms the equivalence of the approaches: the shape parameter estimates are equal, while the scale parameter estimates are related through (4.3).

7.6 Connections with Threshold Excess Model Likelihood

An alternative derivation of the Poisson process model likelihood (7.9) is obtained directly from the threshold excess model of Chapter 4. Let $X_1, \ldots, X_n$ be independent and identically distributed variables. The distribution of the excesses of a high threshold u are assumed to follow a generalized Pareto distribution, with distribution function given by (4.2). Without loss of generality, suppose also that the series $X_1, \ldots, X_n$ corresponds to one year of observations.

Originally, we developed the likelihood for this model by ignoring the X_i that fail to exceed u. We now supplement the likelihood to include partial information on these observations. We first let $\zeta = \Pr\{X_i > u\}$, so that, by (4.6),

$$\zeta = \Pr\{X_i > u\} \approx \frac{1}{n}\left[1 + \xi\left(\frac{u-\mu}{\sigma}\right)\right]^{-1/\xi}, \qquad (7.10)$$

7.6 Connections with Threshold Excess Model Likelihood 135

where (μ, σ, ξ) are the parameters of the corresponding annual maximum GEV distribution. Furthermore, repeating Eq. (4.3),

$$\tilde{\sigma} = \sigma + \xi(u - \mu). \tag{7.11}$$

As we only have a model for the distribution of observations that exceed u, the likelihood contribution of X_i, if it falls below u, is

$$\Pr\{X_i < u\} = 1 - \zeta.$$

On the other hand, for a variable X_i that exceeds u, the likelihood contribution is

$$\Pr\{X_i = x\} = \Pr\{X_i > u\} \Pr\{X_i = x \mid X_i > u\} = \zeta f(x - u; \tilde{\sigma}, \xi),$$

where $f(\cdot; \tilde{\sigma}, \xi)$ denotes the density function of the generalized Pareto distribution with parameters $\tilde{\sigma}$ and ξ. Taking products across the independent observations gives the likelihood

$$L(\zeta, \tilde{\sigma}, \xi; x_1, \ldots, x_n) = (1 - \zeta)^{n - n_u} \prod_{i=1}^{n_u} \zeta \tilde{\sigma}^{-1} \left[1 + \xi \left(\frac{x_i - u}{\tilde{\sigma}} \right) \right]^{-\frac{1}{\xi} - 1}, \tag{7.12}$$

where n_u is the number of exceedances of u. For a high threshold, n_u will be small relative to n, so

$$(1 - \zeta)^{n - n_u} \approx (1 - \zeta)^n \approx \exp\{-n\zeta\}. \tag{7.13}$$

Also,

$$\zeta \tilde{\sigma}^{-1} \left[1 + \xi \left(\frac{x_i - u}{\tilde{\sigma}} \right) \right]^{-\frac{1}{\xi} - 1} =$$

$$(n\tilde{\sigma})^{-1} \left[1 + \xi \left(\frac{x_i - \mu}{\tilde{\sigma}} \right) \right]^{-\frac{1}{\xi} - 1} \times \left[1 + \xi \left(\frac{u - \mu}{\sigma} \right) \right]^{-1/\xi}$$

$$= (n\sigma)^{-1} \left[1 + \xi \left(\frac{x_i - \mu}{\sigma} \right) \right]^{-\frac{1}{\xi} - 1}, \tag{7.14}$$

by (7.10) and repeated use of (7.11). Substituting (7.13) and (7.14) into (7.12) gives, up to proportionality, the likelihood (7.9) with $n_y = 1$. So, apart from the slight approximation at (7.13), the point process likelihood is obtained as the product of the generalized Pareto likelihood for threshold excesses with a likelihood for the binary event of threshold exceedance, reparameterized in terms of the usual GEV parameters.

The equivalence of the limit point process and threshold exceedance model likelihoods confirms that any inference obtained from the point process model could equally have been made within the threshold exceedance

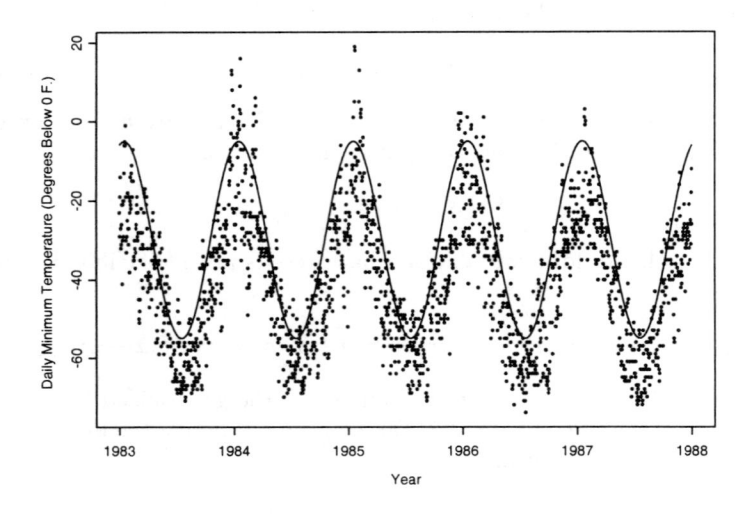

136   7. A Point Process Characterization of Extremes

FIGURE 7.1. Negated Wooster temperature data with time-varying threshold.

framework. The immediate advantages of the point process model are that the natural model parameterization is in terms of the GEV parameters – so that, for example, σ is invariant to threshold – and that the threshold exceedance rate forms part of the inference. These benefits are especially advantageous when the model is adapted to allow for non-stationary effects, by modifying likelihood (7.9) to include temporal or covariate effects in the parameters μ, σ or ξ. In particular, because of the invariance of all parameters to threshold, there is no difficulty in working with models that have time-varying thresholds.

7.7 Wooster Temperature Series

Fig. 7.1 shows the Wooster temperature data again, but now with the addition of a time-varying threshold. Since the parameterization of the point process model is invariant to threshold choice, the only impact of varying a threshold is to affect the bias-variance trade-off in the inference. With such strong seasonal effects as in the Wooster temperature series, it seems sensible to use a threshold that gives an approximately uniform rate of exceedances throughout the year. The threshold shown in Fig. 7.1 was selected by trial-and-error with this objective in mind.

Details of a number of models fitted are given in Table 7.1. The models comprise a time-homogeneous model; periodic models for μ, σ and ξ, so

TABLE 7.1. Number of parameters (p) and maximized log-likelihood (ℓ) for various models fitted to negated Wooster temperature series.

Model	p	ℓ
1. Time-homogeneous	3	−143.6
2. As 1. but periodic in μ	5	126.7
3. As 2. but periodic in $\log \sigma$	7	143.6
4. As 3. but periodic in ξ	9	145.9
5. As 3. plus linear trend in μ and $\log \sigma$	9	145.1
6. As 3. with separate ξ for each season	10	143.9

that, for example,

$$\mu(t) = \beta_0 + \beta_1 \cos(2\pi t/365 - \beta_2),$$

corresponding to a cycle-period of one year; period plus linear trend models; and a model that allows for separate shape parameters in each of the four seasons. As in Chapter 6, the models for σ are specified in terms of $\log \sigma$, so as to preserve positivity on σ.

Judging the log-likelihood values in Table 7.1 relative to the number of parameters in each model, the evidence for periodic effects in μ and σ is overwhelming. That is, likelihood ratio tests comparing models 1, 2 and 3 give strong support for model 3. Comparing models 3 and 4, there is some improvement in allowing a periodic effect in the shape parameter, but the evidence is not conclusive at the 5% level of significance. There is no evidence to support models 4 or 5 – indicating an absence of trend in the extremes – and no reason to adopt a different shape parameter in each of the seasons. Consequently, model 3 is the most appropriate, comprising periodic effects in the location and scale of extremal behavior, but homogeneity in all other aspects. The estimated shape parameter in this model is $\xi = -0.346$, with a standard error of 0.061, implying a reasonably short upper tail to the distribution of extremes across seasons.

The accuracy of the fitted model is supported by residual diagnostic plots shown in Fig. 7.2. These are constructed by transformation of the point process parameter values to the corresponding generalized Pareto parameters, after which the techniques discussed in Chapter 6 are applied directly. Comparing these diagnostics with those of the separate-seasons model in Fig. 6.9, the quality-of-fit of the periodic model is considerably improved.

7.8 Return Level Estimation

For the stationary version of the point process model, return level estimates are easily calculated. For the non-stationary version, calculations

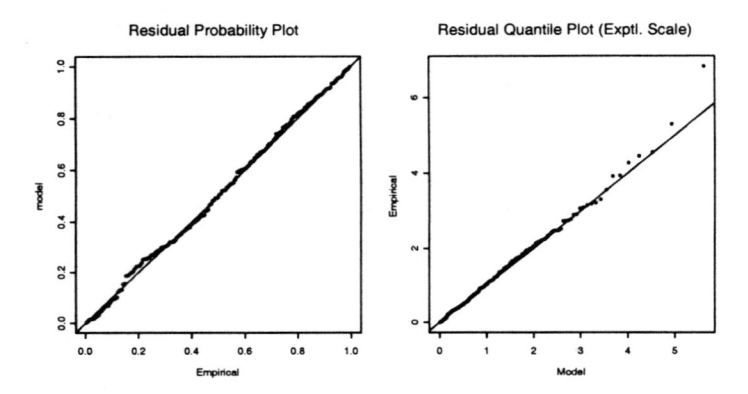

FIGURE 7.2. Diagnostic plots of non-stationary point process model fitted to negated Wooster temperature series.

can still be made, though the precise form depends on the model for non-stationarity. As an example, consider the Wooster temperature model for which there is seasonality over a one-year cycle. Denoting by z_m the m-year return level, and letting n be the number of observations in a year, z_m satisfies the equation

$$1 - \frac{1}{m} = \Pr\{\max(X_1, \ldots, X_n) \leq z_m\} \approx \prod_{i=1}^{n} p_i,$$

where

$$p_i = \begin{cases} 1 - n^{-1}\left[1 + \xi_i(z_m - \mu_i)/\sigma_i\right]^{-1/\xi_i}, & \text{if } [1 + \xi_i(z_m - \mu_i)/\sigma_i] > 0, \\ 1, & \text{otherwise,} \end{cases}$$

and (μ_i, σ_i, ξ_i) are the parameters of the point process model for observation i. Taking logarithms,

$$\sum_{i=1}^{n} \log p_i = \log(1 - 1/m), \tag{7.15}$$

which can easily be solved for z_m using standard numerical methods for non-linear equations.

A difficulty arises in the estimation of standard errors or confidence intervals, since both the delta method and calculation of the profile likelihood

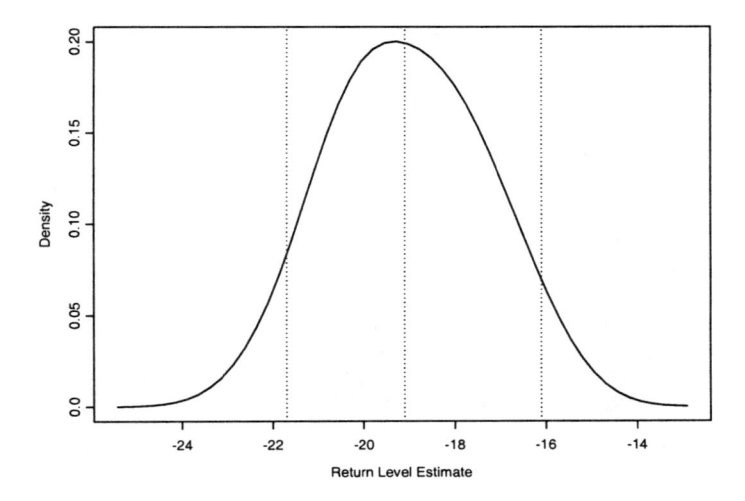

FIGURE 7.3. Approximate sampling distribution of 100-year return level estimate of negated Wooster temperatures. Vertical lines show maximum likelihood estimate and bounds of an approximate 95% confidence interval.

are impractical. A crude approximation can be obtained by simulation. If the sampling distribution of the maximum likelihood estimator of the model parameters were known, we could simulate from this distribution and solve (7.15) for each simulated value, to obtain a realization from the sampling distribution of the return level estimates. Since the sampling distribution is unknown, an alternative is to approximate this procedure by using the multivariate normal approximation (2.9). More precisely, denoting the model parameters by θ, and their maximum likelihood estimate by $\hat{\theta}$, the approximate sampling distribution of the maximum likelihood estimator is $N(\theta, V)$, where V is the estimated variance-covariance matrix.[2] We simulate from this distribution to obtain $\theta_1^*, \ldots, \theta_k^*$, which constitute a sample from the approximate sampling distribution of the maximum likelihood estimator. For each θ_j^*, substitution into (7.15) yields an equation whose solution $z_{m,j}^*$ is a realization from the approximate sampling distribution of $\hat{z}_m$. Finally, the set $z_{m,1}^*, \ldots, z_{m,k}^*$ can be used to construct a density estimate of the distribution, or to obtain approximate confidence intervals.

For the Wooster temperature data, solution of (7.15) based on model 3 leads to an estimate of -19.1 °F for the 100-year return level. Simulation of

---

[2] As usual, it is easier to use the inverse of the observed rather than the expected information matrix.

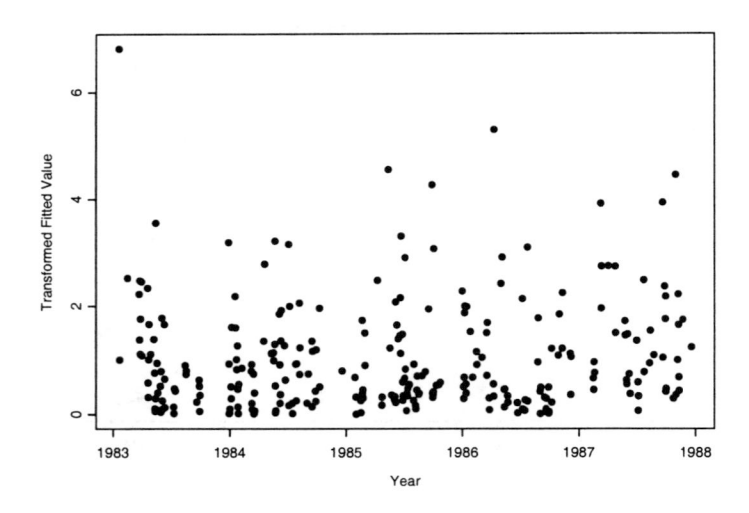

140   7. A Point Process Characterization of Extremes

FIGURE 7.4. Standardized fitted values against time for point process model of negated Wooster temperature series.

the sampling distribution of this estimator led to the smoothed density estimate in Fig. 7.3. This was made on the basis of 100 simulations; improved accuracy would be obtained by increasing the number of simulations, but the procedure is slow because of the requirement to solve (7.15) within each simulation. Added to Fig. 7.3 are lines corresponding to the maximum likelihood estimate and upper and lower bounds of a 95% confidence interval, which turn out to be $[-21.7, -16.1]$.

The estimate and confidence interval indicate some lack-of-fit in this particular example. Within the 5-year observation period the lowest recorded temperature is -19 °F, suggesting it is unlikely that the 100-year return level for negative temperatures is as high as -19.1 °F. Similar problems arise at less extreme levels: the estimated 5-year return level is -13.7 °F, with a 95% confidence interval of $[-16.0, -11.6]$, while there are three recorded temperatures below the value of -14 °F in the five-year span of data.

This issue can be explored further by plotting the standardized fitted values against occurrence time, as in Fig. 7.4. By the model assumptions, the magnitude of the standardized fitted values should be independent of the occurrence time. Fig. 7.4 shows no very obvious departure from this behavior except for a slight tendency for the values to be lower in the winter months. A second complication is dependence in the data. It is clearly seen that large transformed values tend to be closely followed by others, corresponding to nearby extreme values being similar in the original series. This also contradicts the model assumptions. More detailed modeling would be required both to handle the dependence and to better capture the within-year variation.

7.9 r Largest Order Statistic Model

As explained in Section 7.4, Theorems 3.4 and 3.5 can be proved directly from the point process limit representation. Recall that $M_n^{(k)}$ is the kth largest of independent and identically distributed variables $X_1, \ldots, X_n$. Letting
$$N_n = \{(i/(n+1), (X_i - b_n)/a_n) : i = 1, \ldots, n\}$$
and $A_z = (0, 1) \times [z, \infty)$,
$$\Pr\{(M_n^{(k)} - b_n)/a_n \leq z\} = \Pr\{N_n(A_z) \leq k - 1\}$$
$$= \sum_{s=0}^{k-1} \Pr\{N_n(A_z) = s\}. \qquad (7.16)$$

By the Poisson process limit, $N_n(A_z)$ converges, as $n \to \infty$, to a Poisson variable with mean
$$\Lambda(A_z) \left[1 + \xi\left(\frac{z - \mu}{\sigma}\right)\right]^{-1/\xi}.$$

Taking limits in (7.16),
$$\Pr\{(M_n^{(k)} - b_n)/a_n \leq z\} \to \sum_{s=0}^{k-1} e^{-\tau(z)} \frac{\tau(z)^s}{s!},$$
where $\tau(z) = \Lambda(A_z)$. This is Theorem 3.4.

Theorem 3.5 is obtained immediately from the limiting Poisson process likelihood. Let $(z^{(1)}, \ldots, z^{(r)})$ denote the observed value of $\boldsymbol{M}_n$. Substitution of $u = z^{(r)}$, and replacement of the x_i with the $z^{(i)}$ in (7.9), gives the likelihood for the r largest order statistics: Eq. (3.15) in Theorem 3.5.

7.10 Further Reading

General theory on point processes can be found in Cox & Isham (1980). The point process characterization of extremes is originally due to Pickands (1971). The theoretical arguments behind the model are set out in detail by Leadbetter et al. (1983). The potential of the model for direct use in statistical applications was first illustrated by Smith (1989a), whom we have followed closely throughout this chapter. Other applications include Coles & Tawn (1996b), Morton et al. (1997) and Coles & Casson (1999).

8
Multivariate Extremes

8.1 Introduction

In Chapters 3 to 7 we focused on representations and modeling techniques for extremes of a single process. We now turn attention to multivariate extremes. When studying the extremes of two or more processes, each individual process can be modeled using univariate techniques, but there are strong arguments for also studying the extreme value inter-relationships. First, it may be that some combination of the processes is of greater interest than the individual processes themselves; second, in a multivariate model, there is the potential for data on each variable to inform inferences on each of the others. Examples 1.9–1.11 illustrate situations where such techniques may be applicable.

Probability theory for multivariate extremes is well-developed, and there are analogs of the block maximum, threshold and point process results discussed in earlier chapters for univariate extremes. These lead to statistical models, which can again be implemented using likelihood-based techniques. Using such models raises many issues that we have discussed previously in the context of modeling univariate extremes: the models have only an asymptotic justification and their suitability for any particular dataset requires careful checking, for example. But modeling multivariate extremes also raises new issues: the models are less fully prescribed by the general theory and, as with all multivariate models, dimensionality creates difficulties for both model validation and computation. There is an additional problem that some multivariate processes have a strength of dependence that weakens at high levels, to the extent that the most extreme events are near-independent. Traditional methods for multivariate extremes can lead to misleading results for such processes.

In this chapter we give an overview of the various characterizations and models for multivariate extremes. These include versions of the block maxima and threshold excess models for univariate extremes, each of which is a special case of a point process representation. We restrict attention to the two-dimensional, or bivariate, case. This enables us to highlight the main concepts and issues without becoming embroiled in the complexity of notation which a full multivariate treatment would require.

8.2 Componentwise Maxima

8.2.1 Asymptotic Characterization

Suppose that $(X_1, Y_1), (X_2, Y_2) \ldots$ is a sequence of vectors that are independent versions of a random vector having distribution function $F(x, y)$. In an oceanographic setting, (X, Y) might represent pairs of hourly sea-levels at two locations, or values of two sub-components, such as tide and surge levels. As in the univariate case, the classical theory for characterizing the extremal behavior of multivariate extremes is based on the limiting behavior of block maxima. This requires a new definition: with

$$M_{x,n} = \max_{i=1,\ldots,n} \{X_i\} \quad \text{and} \quad M_{y,n} = \max_{i=1,\ldots,n} \{Y_i\},$$

$$\boldsymbol{M}_n = (M_{x,n}, M_{y,n}) \tag{8.1}$$

is the **vector of componentwise maxima**, where the index i, for which the maximum of the X_i sequence occurs, need not be the same as that of the Y_i sequence, so $\boldsymbol{M}_n$ does not necessarily correspond to an observed vector in the original series.

The asymptotic theory of multivariate extremes begins with an analysis of $\boldsymbol{M}_n$ in (8.1), as $n \to \infty$. The issue is partly resolved by recognizing that $\{X_i\}$ and $\{Y_i\}$ considered separately are sequences of independent, univariate random variables. Consequently, standard univariate extreme value results apply to both components. This also means that we can gain some simplicity in presentation by assuming the X_i and Y_i variables to have a known marginal distribution. Other marginal distributions, whose extremal properties are determined by the univariate characterizations, can always be transformed into this standard form. Representations are especially simple if we assume that both X_i and Y_i have the standard Fréchet distribution, with distribution function

$$F(z) = \exp(-1/z), \quad z > 0.$$

144   8. Multivariate Extremes

This is a special case of the GEV distribution with parameters $\mu = 0$, $\sigma = 1$ and $\xi = 1$. By Example 3.2,

$$\Pr\{M_n/n \leq z\} = \exp(-1/z), \quad z > 0, \tag{8.2}$$

which is an exact result for all n because of the max-stability of all members of the GEV family. So, to obtain standard univariate results for each margin, we should consider the re-scaled vector

$$\boldsymbol{M}_n^* = \left(\max_{i=1,\ldots,n}\{X_i\}/n, \max_{i=1,\ldots,n}\{Y_i\}/n\right). \tag{8.3}$$

The following theorem gives a characterization of the limiting joint distribution of $\boldsymbol{M}_n^*$, as $n \to \infty$, providing a bivariate analog of Theorem 3.1.

Theorem 8.1 Let $\boldsymbol{M}_n^* = (M_{x,n}^*, M_{y,n}^*)$ be defined by (8.3), where the (X_i, Y_i) are independent vectors with standard Fréchet marginal distributions. Then if

$$\Pr\{M_{x,n}^* \leq x, M_{y,n}^* \leq y\} \xrightarrow{d} G(x,y), \tag{8.4}$$

where G is a non-degenerate distribution function, G has the form

$$G(x,y) = \exp\{-V(x,y)\}, \quad x > 0, \ y > 0 \tag{8.5}$$

where

$$V(x,y) = 2\int_0^1 \max\left(\frac{w}{x}, \frac{1-w}{y}\right) dH(w), \tag{8.6}$$

and H is a distribution function on $[0,1]$ satisfying the mean constraint

$$\int_0^1 w\,dH(w) = 1/2. \tag{8.7}$$

□

The family of distributions that arise as limits in (8.4) is termed the class of **bivariate extreme value distributions**. Theorem 8.1 implies that this class is in one-one correspondence with the set of distribution functions H on $[0,1]$ satisfying (8.7). If H is differentiable with density h, integral (8.6) is simply

$$V(x,y) = 2\int_0^1 \max\left(\frac{w}{x}, \frac{1-w}{y}\right) h(w)\,dw.$$

However, bivariate extreme value distributions are also generated by measures H that are not differentiable. For example, when H is a measure that places mass 0.5 on $w = 0$ and $w = 1$, (8.7) is trivially satisfied,

$$V(x,y) = x^{-1} + y^{-1}$$

by (8.6), and the corresponding bivariate extreme value distribution is

$$G(x,y) = \exp\{-(x^{-1} + y^{-1})\}, \quad x > 0, \ y > 0.$$

This function factorizes across x and y, and therefore corresponds to independent variables. Similarly, if H is a measure that places unit mass on $w = 0.5$, (8.7) is again satisfied trivially, and the corresponding bivariate extreme value distribution is

$$G(x,y) = \exp\{-\max(x^{-1}, y^{-1})\}, \quad x > 0, \ y > 0.$$

which is the distribution function of variables that are marginally standard Fréchet, but which are perfectly dependent: $X = Y$ with probability 1.

Since the GEV family provides the complete class of marginal limit distributions, it follows that the complete class of bivariate limits is obtained simply by generalizing the marginal distributions. Specifically, letting

$$\tilde{x} = \left[1 + \xi_x \left(\frac{x - \mu_x}{\sigma_x}\right)\right]^{1/\xi_x} \quad \text{and} \quad \tilde{y} = \left[1 + \xi_y \left(\frac{y - \mu_y}{\sigma_y}\right)\right]^{1/\xi_y},$$

the complete family of bivariate extreme value distributions, with arbitrary GEV margins, has distribution function of the form

$$G(x,y) = \exp\left\{-V(\tilde{x}, \tilde{y})\right\}, \tag{8.8}$$

provided $[1 + \xi_x(x - \mu_x)/\sigma_x] > 0$ and $[1 + \xi_y(y - \mu_y)/\sigma_y] > 0$, and where the function V satisfies (8.6) for some choice of H. The marginal distributions are GEV with parameters (μ_x, σ_x, ξ_x) and (μ_y, σ_y, ξ_y) respectively.

It is easy to check from (8.6) that, for any constant $a > 0$,

$$V\left(a^{-1}x, a^{-1}y\right) = aV(x,y);$$

V is said to be **homogeneous of order** -1. Using this property in (8.5), we obtain

$$G^n(x,y) = G\left(n^{-1}x, n^{-1}y\right), \tag{8.9}$$

for $n = 2, 3, \ldots$, so if (X, Y) has distribution function G, then $\boldsymbol{M}_n$ also has distribution function G, apart from a re-scaling by n^{-1}. Therefore, G possesses a multivariate version of the property of max-stability introduced in Chapter 3. An argument similar to that of Chapter 3 implies that limit distributions in (8.4) must have this property of max-stability, and, like in the univariate case, this argument forms the basis of a proof of Theorem 8.1 (Resnick, 1987, for example). That is, from (8.9), distributions of the type (8.5) have the property of max-stability, and can be shown to be the only distributions having this property, subject to the marginal specification.

Although Theorem 8.1 provides a complete characterization of bivariate limit distributions, the class of possible limits is wide, being constrained only by (8.6). In particular, any distribution function H on $[0,1]$ in (8.6), satisfying the mean constraint (8.7), gives rise to a valid limit in (8.4). This leads to difficulties, as the limit family has no finite parameterization. One possibility is to use nonparametric methods of estimation, but this is also complicated by the fact that it is not straightforward to constrain nonparametric estimators to satisfy functional constraints of the type (8.7). An alternative is to use parametric sub-families of distributions for H, leading to sub-families of distributions for G. In this way, only a small subset of the complete class of limit distributions for G is obtained, but by careful choice it is possible to ensure that a wide sub-class of the entire limit family is approximated. Put another way, we can obtain parametric families for H, and hence G, such that every member of the full limit class for G can be closely approximated by a member of the sub-family generated by the family of H. In principle it is simple to build models: we just require a parametric family for H on $[0,1]$ whose mean is equal to 0.5 for every value of the parameter. Substitution into (8.6) and (8.5) then generates the corresponding family for G. In practice it is not so easy to generate parametric families whose mean is parameter-free, and for which the integral in (8.6) is tractable.

One standard class is the logistic family:

$$G(x,y) = \exp\left\{-\left(x^{-1/\alpha} + y^{-1/\alpha}\right)^\alpha\right\}, \quad x > 0,\ y > 0, \qquad (8.10)$$

for a parameter $\alpha \in (0,1)$. The derivation from (8.6) is not obvious, but it can be shown that (8.10) is obtained by letting H have the density function

$$h(w) = \frac{1}{2}(\alpha^{-1} - 1)\{w(1-w)\}^{-1-1/\alpha}\{w^{-1/\alpha} + (1-w)^{-1/\alpha}\}^{\alpha-2} \qquad (8.11)$$

on $0 < w < 1$. The mean constraint (8.7) is automatically satisfied for this model because of symmetry about $w = 0.5$.

The main reason for the popularity of the logistic family is its flexibility. As $\alpha \to 1$ in (8.10),

$$G(x,y) \to \exp\left\{-(x^{-1} + y^{-1})\right\},$$

corresponding to independent variables; as $\alpha \to 0$,

$$G(x,y) \to \exp\left\{-\max(x^{-1}, y^{-1})\right\},$$

corresponding to perfectly dependent variables. Hence, the sub-family of bivariate extreme value distributions generated by the logistic family covers all levels of dependence from independence to perfect dependence. A limitation of the logistic model is that the variables x and y in (8.10) are exchangeable. This arises because of the symmetry of the density h. Although this is the easiest way to guarantee that the mean constraint is satisfied, models generated in this way are bound to be exchangeable in the component variables.

A generalization of the logistic model that allows for asymmetry in the dependence structure is the **bilogistic model**, derived by Joe et al. (1992). This is obtained by letting H have the density function

$$h(w) = \frac{1}{2}(1-\alpha)(1-w)^{-1}w^{-2}(1-u)u^{1-\alpha}\{\alpha(1-u)+\beta u\}^{-1}$$

on $0 < w < 1$, where α and β are parameters such that $0 < \alpha < 1$ and $0 < \beta < 1$, and $u = u(w, \alpha, \beta)$ is the solution of

$$(1-\alpha)(1-w)(1-u)^\beta - (1-\beta)wu^\alpha = 0.$$

In the special case that $\alpha = \beta$, the bilogistic model reduces to the logistic model. More generally, the value of $\alpha - \beta$ determines the extent of asymmetry in the dependence structure.

An alternative asymmetric model, proposed by Coles & Tawn (1991), is the **Dirichlet model**,[1] for which

$$h(w) = \frac{\alpha\beta\Gamma(\alpha+\beta+1)(\alpha w)^{\alpha-1}\{\beta(1-w)\}^{\beta-1}}{2\Gamma(\alpha)\Gamma(\beta)\{\alpha w + \beta(1-w)\}^{\alpha+\beta+1}}$$

on $0 < w < 1$, where the parameters satisfy $\alpha > 0$ and $\beta > 0$. Like the bilogistic model, the Dirichlet model is symmetric only in the case $\alpha = \beta$.

8.2.2 Modeling

Theorem 8.1 can be put into practice in the following way. From an original series $(x_1, y_1), \ldots, (x_n, y_n)$ of independent vectors we form a sequence of componentwise block maxima $(z_{1,1}, z_{2,1}), \ldots, (z_{1,m}, z_{2,m})$. Choice of block size involves the same considerations of bias and variance as in the univariate case. Again, a pragmatic choice is often made; typically, a block length corresponding to one year of observations.

Considered separately, the series $z_{1,1} \ldots, z_{1,m}$ and $z_{2,1}, \ldots, z_{2,m}$ are sequences of independent block maxima that can be individually modeled using the GEV distribution; i.e. for each j, $z_{i,j}$ is treated as an independent realization of a random variable Z_i, for $i = 1, 2$, where

$$Z_i \sim \text{GEV}(\mu_i, \sigma_i, \xi_i).$$

Applying maximum likelihood to the separate series generates estimates, denoted $(\hat{\mu}_i, \hat{\sigma}_i, \hat{\xi}_i)$, for $i = 1, 2$. The transformed variable

$$\tilde{Z}_i = \left[1 + \hat{\xi}_i \left(\frac{Z_i - \hat{\mu}_i}{\hat{\sigma}_i}\right)\right]^{1/\hat{\xi}_i} \tag{8.12}$$

---

[1] The name Dirichlet is used since the model is developed by transformation of the standard Dirichlet family of distributions; the nomenclature is not intended to imply that the two families are identical.

TABLE 8.1. Maximum likelihood estimates (MLE) and standard errors (SE) for logistic model fitted to bivariate series of annual maximum sea-levels at Fremantle and Port Pirie.

	Fremantle			Port Pirie			
	μ_x	σ_x	ξ_x	μ_y	σ_y	ξ_y	α
MLE	1.51	0.117	−0.149	3.87	0.197	−0.043	0.922
SE	0.02	0.012	0.093	0.03	0.021	0.100	0.087

is therefore approximately distributed according to the standard Fréchet distribution. The pairs $(\tilde{z}_{1,j}, \tilde{z}_{2,j})$, obtained by substituting the observations $(z_{1,j}, z_{2,j})$ into (8.12), comprise a sequence of independent realizations of a vector having bivariate extreme value distribution within the family (8.5). The probability density function of this model is

$$g(x,y) = \{V_x(x,y)V_y(x,y) - V_{xy}(x,y)\}\exp\{-V(x,y)\}, \quad x > 0,\ y > 0,$$

where V_x, V_y and $V_{x,y}$ denote partial and mixed derivatives of V respectively. Assuming a model for V with parameter θ, such as that provided by the logistic model with $\theta = \alpha$, leads to the likelihood

$$L(\theta) = \prod_{i=1}^{m} g(\tilde{z}_{1,i}, \tilde{z}_{2,i}), \tag{8.13}$$

and the corresponding log-likelihood

$$\ell(\theta) = \sum_{i=1}^{m} \log g(\tilde{z}_{1,i}, \tilde{z}_{2,i}).$$

Standard techniques yield maximum likelihood estimates and standard errors of θ.

Equation (8.13) can also be regarded as a full likelihood for marginal and dependence parameters, taking g to be the density of (8.8) rather than (8.5). This procedure combines the transformation and maximization into a single step, enabling a potential gain in efficiency due to the transfer of information across variables. The price for the gain in statistical efficiency is an increase in the computational cost.

8.2.3 Example: Annual Maximum Sea-levels

Fig. 8.1 shows the annual maximum sea-level at Port Pirie, against the corresponding value at Fremantle, for years in which both values were recorded. There seems to be a slight tendency for large values of one variable to correspond to large values of the other, though the effect is not strong. Assuming the logistic model and using the two-stage estimation procedure

8.2 Componentwise Maxima 149

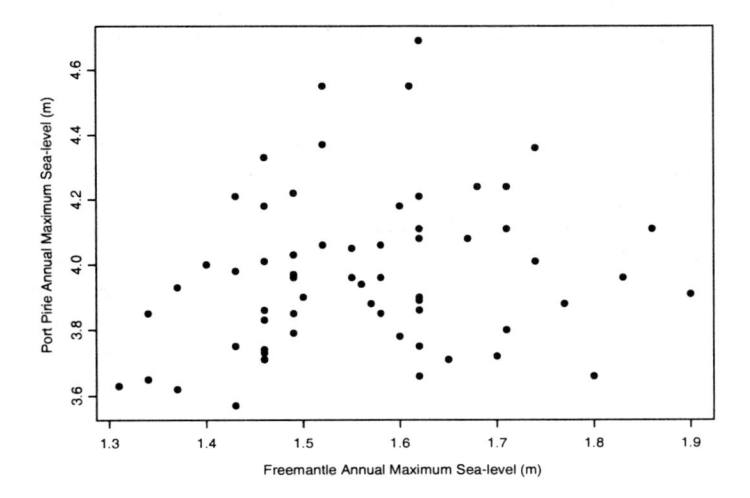

FIGURE 8.1. Annual maximum sea-levels at Fremantle and Port Pirie.

– first estimating the marginal distributions, and then the joint distribution after marginal transformation – yields the results in Table 8.1. The marginal parameter estimates are similar to those obtained for these variables in earlier chapters, the slight differences arising because the bivariate analysis is restricted to years in which both sites have data. The logistic dependence parameter estimate is $\hat{\alpha} = 0.922$, corresponding to weak dependence. Stronger dependence in extreme sea-levels is likely for sites that are geographically closer than the two studied here.

A number of modifications could be made to the analysis. First, since additional data from the individual sites are available for years in which the value from the other site is missing, it may be preferable to apply the marginal estimation to the extended series, and use these estimates to transform the bivariate data prior to joint distribution estimation. Better still, if a joint likelihood is used to simultaneously estimate marginal and dependence parameters, the log-likelihood can be written

$$\ell(\theta) = \sum_{I_{1,2}} \log g(z_{1,i}, z_{2,i}) + \sum_{I_1} \log g_1(z_{1,i}) + \sum_{I_2} \log g_2(z_{2,i}), \quad (8.14)$$

where $I_{1,2}, I_1$ and I_2 denote the indexes of years in which, respectively, both, only the first, and only the second, sites have data, and g_1 and g_2 are the marginal densities of g. Maximizing (8.14) corresponds to an analysis in which all the available information is utilized and the potential for sharing information across sites is exploited. A second modification is to allow for possible non-stationarity in either or both variables. As in Chapter 6, this is handled by enabling time variation in any of the individual model parameters. For this particular example, as we saw in Chapter 6, there is an apparent linear trend in the Fremantle data, so that the substitution of

$$\mu(t) = \alpha + \beta t$$

in the appropriate likelihood should lead to an improved analysis. Again, this can either be done as part of a preliminary marginal analysis, in which case the marginal transformation (8.12) will also be time-dependent, or it can be incorporated into a full likelihood of the type (8.14). Finally, it is possible to exploit commonality of distributional aspects across variables. For example, it may be that while the GEV parameters μ and σ are different at the two locations, due to different local features such as topography and bathymetry, the parameter ξ is globally determined by large-scale features of the sea-level process. It may therefore be desirable to impose the constraint $\xi_1 = \xi_2$, or at least, to examine the evidence in support of such a model reduction. This cannot be achieved with the two-stage procedure, requiring instead a single model likelihood of the form (8.14). The strength of evidence for the model reduction is obtained from a standard likelihood ratio test, comparing the maximized log-likelihoods of models with, and without, the constraint $\xi_1 = \xi_2$.

8.2.4 Structure Variables

To simplify notation, we now denote the componentwise maxima vector by $\boldsymbol{M} = (M_x, M_y)$, ignoring the implicit dependence on the block size n. Although inference may be carried out on replicate observations of $\boldsymbol{M}$, corresponding, perhaps, to a series of componentwise annual maxima, it may be the extremal behavior of some combination of the variables,

$$Z = \phi(M_x, M_y),$$

that is of more interest. In this context, Z is termed a **structure variable**. Possibilities for Z include $\max\{M_x, M_y\}$, $\min\{M_x, M_y\}$ or $M_x + M_y$. Denoting the probability density function of (M_x, M_y) by g, the distribution function of Z is

$$\Pr\{Z \leq z\} = \int_{A_z} g(x, y) dx dy, \qquad (8.15)$$

where $A_z = \{(x, y) : \phi(x, y) \leq z\}$. For some choices of ϕ, the integration can be avoided. For example, if $Z = \max\{M_x, M_y\}$,

$$\Pr\{Z \leq z\} = \Pr\{M_x \leq z, M_y \leq z\} = G(z, z), \qquad (8.16)$$

where G is the joint distribution function of $\boldsymbol{M}$.

The N-year return level of a structure variable Z is the solution of

$$G_Z(z) = 1 - 1/N, \qquad (8.17)$$

8.2 Componentwise Maxima

where G_Z is the distribution function of Z. This can be complicated to obtain if the distribution function is given only in integral form (8.15). In simpler cases, such as (8.16), the solution of (8.17) is likely to be straightforward using standard numerical techniques. The calculation of standard errors or confidence intervals is less straightforward, but we can use the technique of simulating the approximate sampling distribution using the approximate normality of the maximum likelihood estimator, as described in Section 7.8.

An alternative, and much simpler, procedure for estimating return levels of a structure variable $Z = \phi(M_x, M_y)$ is based on univariate techniques. Given the series of componentwise maxima $(m_{x,1}, m_{y,1}), \ldots, (m_{x,k}, m_{y,k})$, where each observation $(m_{x,i}, m_{y,i})$ is a realization of the random vector M, we can form the series $z_1, \ldots, z_k$, where $z_i = \phi(m_{x,i}, m_{y,i})$. Assuming the z_i to be realizations from a GEV distribution, standard univariate modeling techniques can be used to estimate the distribution and to calculate return levels. This approach is sometimes referred to as the **structure variable method**. Offsetting its simplicity, there are a number of disadvantages. First, the justification for the GEV model is not strong: if the entire dataset were available, and not just the annual maxima, it is possible that applying ϕ to an individual pair may generate a larger value than applying ϕ to the annual maxima of X and Y. Second, the method does not enable the inclusion of data for periods when one of the variables is missing. Finally, the method requires a separate analysis for each choice of structure variable.

We can compare the structure variable and bivariate procedures using the Fremantle and Port Pirie annual maximum sea-level data. We denote by (M_x, M_y) the componentwise annual maximum sea-levels at Fremantle and Port Pirie respectively, and use the logistic analysis reported in Table 8.1. The variable $Z = \max\{M_x, M_y\}$ is of little interest here, since the difference in mean levels at the two locations means that the Port Pirie value is always greater than the Fremantle value. As an illustration, we therefore consider

$$Z = \max\{M_x, (M_y - 2.5)\},$$

which is the larger of the two annual maxima after a 2.5 m approximate correction for differences in mean sea-level. The bivariate analysis leads to the return level plot in Fig. 8.2, with 95% confidence intervals obtained by the simulation technique.

A comparison with the structure variable analysis is given in Fig. 8.3. In this particular example, there is little difference between the two estimated return level curves, and both seem to give a faithful representation of the empirical estimates provided by the empirical distribution function of the z_i. The widths of the confidence intervals are also similar, although those based on the bivariate analysis reflect better the greater uncertainty at the upper end of the interval.

152   8. Multivariate Extremes

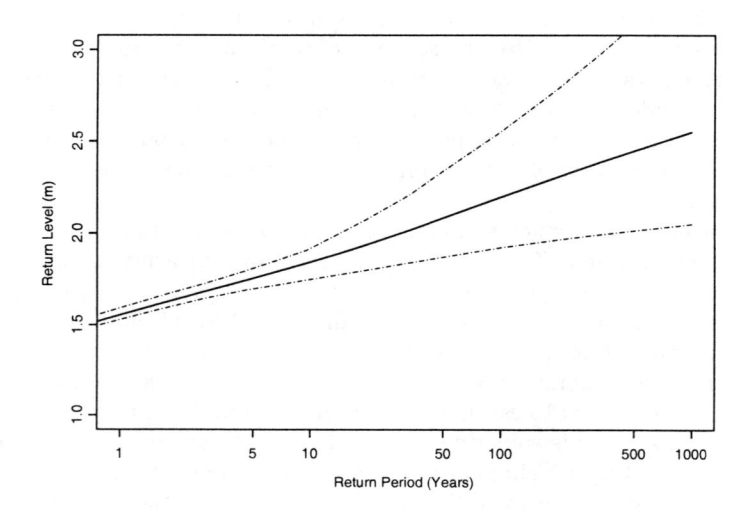

FIGURE 8.2. Return level plot with 95% confidence intervals for $Z = \max\{M_x, (M_y - 2.5)\}$ in Fremantle and Port Pirie annual maximum sea-level analysis.

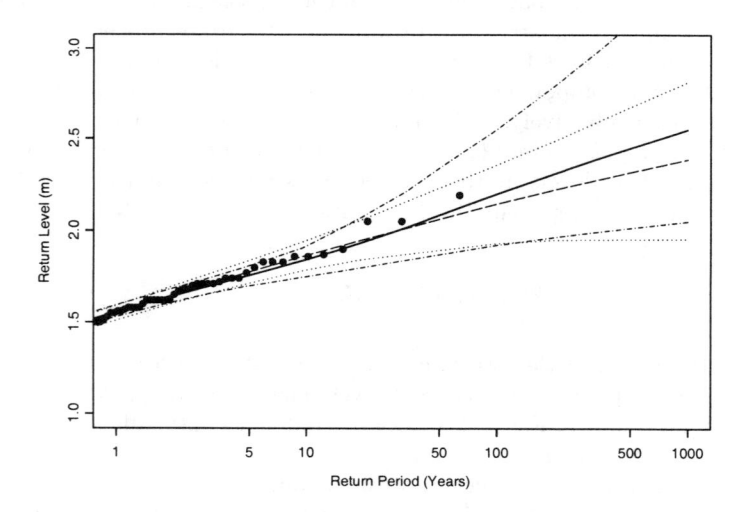

FIGURE 8.3. Comparison of return level plots and 95% confidence intervals for $Z = \max\{M_x, (M_y - 2.5)\}$ in Fremantle and Port Pirie annual maximum sea-level analysis. Solid line corresponds to bivariate analysis, with 95% confidence intervals given as the dot-dashed line. Dashed line corresponds to structure variable analysis with 95% confidence intervals given as dotted lines. Points correspond to empirical estimates based on the observed z_i.

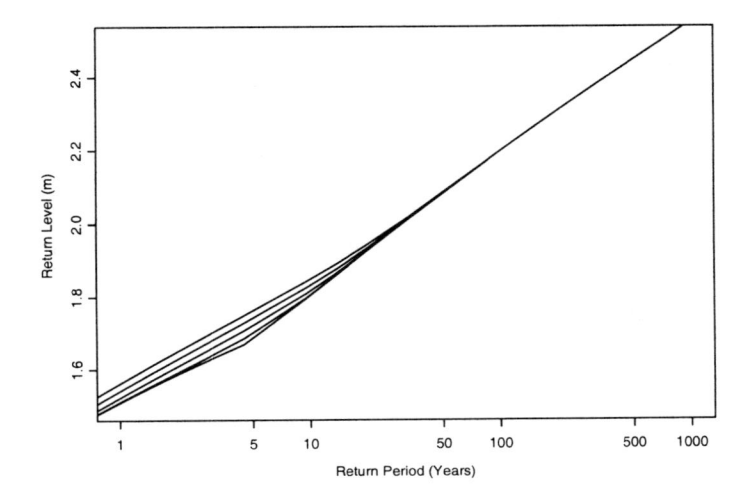

FIGURE 8.4. Comparison of return level plot for $Z = \max\{M_x, (M_y - 2.5)\}$ in logistic model analysis of Fremantle and Port Pirie annual maximum sea-level series with $\alpha = 0$, 0.25, 0.5, 0.75, 1 respectively. Lowest curve corresponds to $\alpha = 0$; highest to $\alpha = 1$.

The impact of dependence can be explored by plotting the return level curve obtained from models with the estimated marginal parameter values, but paired with a range of values of the dependence parameter α. For the bivariate sea-level analysis with $Z = \max\{M_x, (M_y - 2.5)\}$ in the sea-level example in Fig. 8.4 it emerges that different dependence parameter values have little effect on the value of return levels, so there is little to be gained in precise modeling of dependence if Z is the structure variable of interest. However, other quantities are likely to be affected to a greater extent. For example, Fig. 8.5 shows the corresponding plot for the structure variable $\tilde{Z} = \min\{M_x, (M_y - 2.5)\}$. In this case, particularly at extreme levels, substantially different return levels are obtained for different parameter values, and especially so when $\alpha \approx 1$. So, while inferences on some variables are robust to dependence assumptions, others are more sensitive.

8.3 Alternative Representations

There are alternative representations of multivariate extreme value behavior that avoid the wastefulness of data implied by an analysis of componentwise block maxima. In particular, analogs of the univariate threshold

154   8. Multivariate Extremes

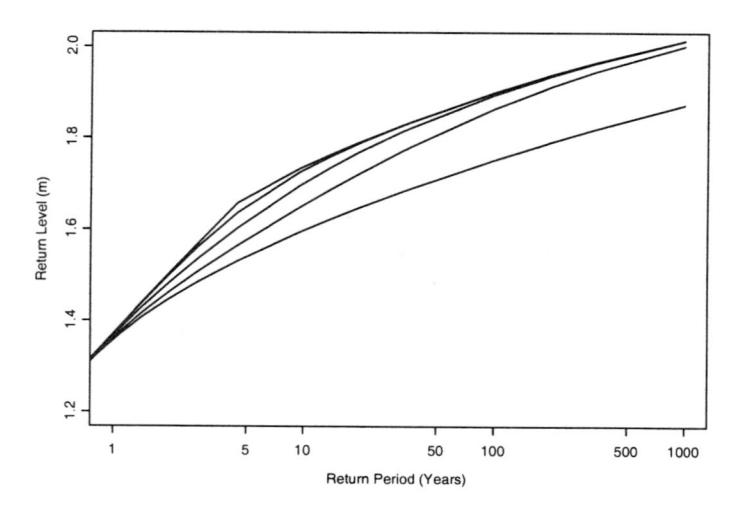

FIGURE 8.5. Comparison of return level plot for $Z = \min\{M_x, (M_y - 2.5)\}$ in logistic model analysis of Fremantle and Port Pirie annual maximum sea-level series with $\alpha = 0$, 0.25, 0.5, 0.75 and 1, respectively. Lowest curve corresponds to $\alpha = 1$; highest to $\alpha = 0$.

excess model and point process model can be obtained. In this section we give a brief description of both techniques.

8.3.1 Bivariate Threshold Excess Model

In Chapter 4 we derived as a class of approximations to the tail of an arbitrary distribution function F the family

$$G(x) = 1 - \zeta\left\{1 + \frac{\xi(x-u)}{\sigma}\right\}^{-1/\xi}, \quad x > u. \quad (8.18)$$

This means there are parameters ζ, σ and ξ such that, for a large enough threshold u, $F(x) \approx G(x)$ on $x > u$. Our aim now is to obtain a bivariate version of (8.18), i.e. a family with which to approximate an arbitrary joint distribution $F(x,y)$ on regions of the form $x > u_x, y > u_y$, for large enough u_x and u_y.

Suppose $(x_1, y_1), \ldots, (x_n, y_n)$ are independent realizations of a random variable (X, Y) with joint distribution function F. For suitable thresholds u_x and u_y, the marginal distributions of F each have an approximation of the form (8.18), with respective parameter sets $(\zeta_x, \sigma_x, \xi_x)$ and $(\zeta_y, \sigma_y, \xi_y)$.

The transformations

$$\tilde{X} = -\left(\log\left\{1 - \zeta_x\left[1 + \frac{\xi_x(X - u_x)}{\sigma_x}\right]^{-1/\xi_x}\right\}\right)^{-1} \quad (8.19)$$

and

$$\tilde{Y} = -\left(\log\left\{1 - \zeta_y\left[1 + \frac{\xi_y(Y - u_y)}{\sigma_y}\right]^{-1/\xi_y}\right\}\right)^{-1} \quad (8.20)$$

induce a variable $(\tilde{X}, \tilde{Y})$ whose distribution function $\tilde{F}$ has margins that are approximately standard Fréchet for $X > u_x$ and $Y > u_y$. By (8.5), for large n,

$$\begin{aligned}\tilde{F}(\tilde{x}, \tilde{y}) &= \left\{\tilde{F}^n(\tilde{x}, \tilde{y})\right\}^{1/n} \\ &\approx [\exp\{-V(\tilde{x}/n, \tilde{y}/n)\}]^{1/n} \\ &= \exp\{-V(\tilde{x}, \tilde{y})\},\end{aligned}$$

because of the homogeneity property of V. Finally, since $F(x, y) = \tilde{F}(\tilde{x}, \tilde{y})$, it follows that

$$F(x, y) \approx G(x, y) = \exp\{-V(\tilde{x}, \tilde{y})\}, \quad x > u_x, y > u_y, \quad (8.21)$$

with $\tilde{x}$ and $\tilde{y}$ defined in terms of x and y by (8.19) and (8.20). This assumes that the thresholds u_x and u_y are large enough to justify the limit (8.5) as an approximation. We discuss this point further in Section 8.4.

Inference for this model is complicated by the fact that a bivariate pair may exceed a specified threshold in just one of its components. Let

$$R_{0,0} = (-\infty, u_x) \times (-\infty, u_y), R_{1,0} = [u_x, \infty) \times (-\infty, u_y),$$
$$R_{0,1} = (-\infty, u_x) \times [u_y, \infty), R_{1,1} = [u_x, \infty) \times [u_y, \infty),$$

so that, for example, a point $(x, y) \in R_{1,0}$ if the x-component exceeds the threshold u_x, but the y-component is below u_y. For points in $R_{1,1}$, model (8.21) applies, and the density of $\tilde{F}$ gives the appropriate likelihood component. On the other regions, since $\tilde{F}$ is not applicable, it is necessary to censor the likelihood component. For example, suppose that $(x, y) \in R_{1,0}$. Then since $x > u_x$, but $y < u_y$, there is information in the data concerning the marginal x-component, but not the y-component. Hence, the likelihood contribution for such a point is

$$\Pr\{X = x, Y \leq u_y\} = \left.\frac{\partial F}{\partial x}\right|_{(x, u_y)}$$

as this is the only information in the datum concerning F. Applying similar considerations in the other regions, we obtain the likelihood function

$$L(\theta; (x_1, y_1), \ldots, (x_n, y_n)) = \prod_{i=1}^{n} \psi(\theta; (x_i, y_i)), \quad (8.22)$$

where θ denotes the parameters of F and

$$\psi(\theta;(x,y)) = \begin{cases} \left.\frac{\partial^2 F}{\partial x \partial y}\right|_{(x,y)} & \text{if } (x,y) \in R_{1,1}, \\ \left.\frac{\partial F}{\partial x}\right|_{(x,u_y)} & \text{if } (x,y) \in R_{1,0}, \\ \left.\frac{\partial F}{\partial y}\right|_{(u_x,y)} & \text{if } (x,y) \in R_{0,1}, \\ F(u_x, u_y) & \text{if } (x,y) \in R_{0,0}, \end{cases}$$

with each term being derived from the joint tail approximation (8.21). Maximizing the log-likelihood leads to estimates and standard errors for the parameters of F in the usual way. As with the componentwise block maxima model, the inference can be simplified by carrying out the marginal estimation, followed by transformations (8.19) and (8.20), as a preliminary step. In this case, likelihood (8.22) is a function only of the dependence parameters contained in the model for V.

An alternative method, if there is a natural structure variable $Z = \phi(X, Y)$, is to apply univariate threshold techniques to the series $z_i = \phi(x_i, y_i)$. This approach now makes more sense, since the z_i are functions of concurrent events. In terms of statistical efficiency, however, there are still good reasons to prefer the multivariate model.

8.3.2 Point Process Model

The point process characterization, summarized by the following theorem, includes an interpretation of the function H in (8.6).

Theorem 8.2 Let $(x_1, y_1), (x_2, y_2) \ldots$ be a sequence of independent bivariate observations from a distribution with standard Fréchet margins that satisfies the convergence for componentwise maxima

$$\Pr\{M_{x,n}^* \leq x, M_{y,n}^* \leq y\} \to G(x,y).$$

Let $\{N_n\}$ be a sequence of point processes defined by

$$N_n = \{(n^{-1}x_1, n^{-1}y_1), \ldots, (n^{-1}x_n, n^{-1}y_n)\}. \tag{8.23}$$

Then,

$$N_n \xrightarrow{d} N$$

on regions bounded from the origin $(0,0)$, where N is a non-homogeneous Poisson process on $(0, \infty) \times (0, \infty)$. Moreover, letting

$$r = x + y \quad \text{and} \quad w = \frac{x}{x+y}, \tag{8.24}$$

the intensity function of N is

$$\lambda(r, w) = 2\frac{dH(w)}{r^2}, \tag{8.25}$$

where H is related to G through (8.5) and (8.6). □

To interpret this result it is necessary to understand the effect of the transformations defined by (8.24): $(x, y) \to (r, w)$ is a transformation from Cartesian to pseudo-polar coordinates, in which r gives a measure of distance from the origin and w measures angle on a $[0, 1]$ scale. In particular, $w = 0$ and $w = 1$ correspond to the $x = 0$ and $y = 0$ axes respectively. Equation (8.25) then implies that the intensity of the limiting process N factorizes across radial and angular components. In other words, the angular spread of points of N is determined by H, and is independent of radial distance. The mysterious appearance of H in (8.6) is explained by its role in determining the angular spread of points in the limit Poisson process. Interpretation is easiest if H is differentiable, with density h. Then, since w measures the relative size of the (x, y) pair, $h(\cdot)$ determines the relative frequency of events of different relative size. If extremes are near-independent, we would expect large values of x/n to occur with small values of y/n, and vice versa. In this case, $h(w)$ is large close to $w = 0$ and $w = 1$, and small elsewhere. In contrast, if dependence is very strong, so that x/n and y/n are likely to be similar in value, $h(w)$ is large close to $w = 1/2$. The reason for maintaining the greater generality in (8.25), rather than assuming that H always has a density h, is to allow for two special limit cases. First, when G corresponds to independent variables, the measure function H comprises atoms of mass 0.5 on $w = 0$ and $w = 1$; second, when G corresponds to perfectly dependent variables, H consists of an atom of unit mass at $w = 0.5$.

As in the univariate case, all multivariate representations can be derived as special cases of the point process representation. We illustrate this by deriving the limit distribution of componentwise block maxima. Using the notation of Theorem 8.1,

$$\Pr\{M^*_{x,n} \le x, M^*_{y,n} \le y\} = \Pr\{N_n(A) = 0\},$$

where N_n is the point process defined by (8.23) and

$$A = \{(0, \infty) \times (0, \infty)\} \setminus \{(0, x) \times (0, y)\}.$$

So, by the Poisson process limit,

$$\Pr\{M^*_{x,n} \le x, M^*_{y,n} \le y\} \to \Pr\{N(A) = 0\} = \exp\{-\Lambda(A)\}, \qquad (8.26)$$

where

$$\begin{aligned}
\Lambda(A) &= \int_A 2\frac{dr}{r^2} dH(w) \\
&= \int_{w=0}^1 \int_{r=\min\{x/w, y/(1-w)\}}^\infty 2\frac{dr}{r^2} dH(w) \\
&= 2\int_{w=0}^1 \max\left(\frac{w}{x}, \frac{1-w}{y}\right) dH(w). \qquad (8.27)
\end{aligned}$$

Putting together (8.26) and (8.27) gives Theorem 8.1.

To use the point process characterization in practice, we assume the Poisson limit to be a reasonable approximation to N_n on an appropriate region. Convergence is guaranteed on regions bounded from the origin. Things are especially simple if we choose a region of the type $A = \{(x,y) : x/n + y/n > r_0\}$, for suitably large r_0, since then

$$\Lambda(A) = 2\int_A \frac{dr}{r^2} dH(w) = 2\int_{r=r_0}^{\infty} \frac{dr}{r^2} \int_{w=0}^{1} dH(w) = 2/r_0,$$

which is constant with respect to the parameters of H. Hence, assuming H has density h,

$$\begin{aligned} L(\theta; (x_1, y_1), \ldots, (x_n, y_n)) &= \exp\{-\Lambda(A)\} \prod_{i=1}^{N_A} \lambda(x_{(i)}/n, y_{(i)}/n) \\ &\propto \prod_{i=1}^{N_A} h(w_i), \end{aligned} \quad (8.28)$$

where $w_i = x_{(i)}/(x_{(i)} + y_{(i)})$ for the N_A points $(x_{(i)}, y_{(i)})$ falling in A. This assumes that the data $(x_1, y_1), \ldots, (x_n, y_n)$ have marginal standard Fréchet distributions. We can arrange this by marginal estimation and transformation prior to dependence modeling. Joint estimation of marginal and dependence parameters is also possible, though the likelihood is substantially more complicated.

8.3.3 Examples

We illustrate the bivariate threshold excess and point process models with the oceanographic data of Example 1.10 and the exchange rate data of Example 1.11. For simplicity of presentation, we show only the two-stage analyses, in which the data are modeled marginally and transformed to standard Fréchet variables prior to dependence modeling.

After transformation to standard Fréchet variables, the wave and surge data of Example 1.10 are plotted on logarithmic scales in Fig. 8.6. Marginal thresholds corresponding to the 95% marginal quantiles have also been added. With these thresholds, and assuming the logistic model, maximization of likelihood (8.22) leads to an estimate of $\hat{\alpha} = 0.758$, with a standard error of 0.026. This corresponds to a model with a reasonably weak level of dependence, but which is significantly different from independence.

Analysis of the same data using the point process model requires the specification of a threshold u to determine the points which contribute to the likelihood (8.28). For comparison with the threshold analysis, we choose u such that the intersection of the threshold with the axes occurs at the same points as in Fig. 8.6. On a Fréchet scale, the threshold boundary is chosen so that $X + Y = r_0$ for some value of r_0. After log-transformation,

8.3 Alternative Representations 159

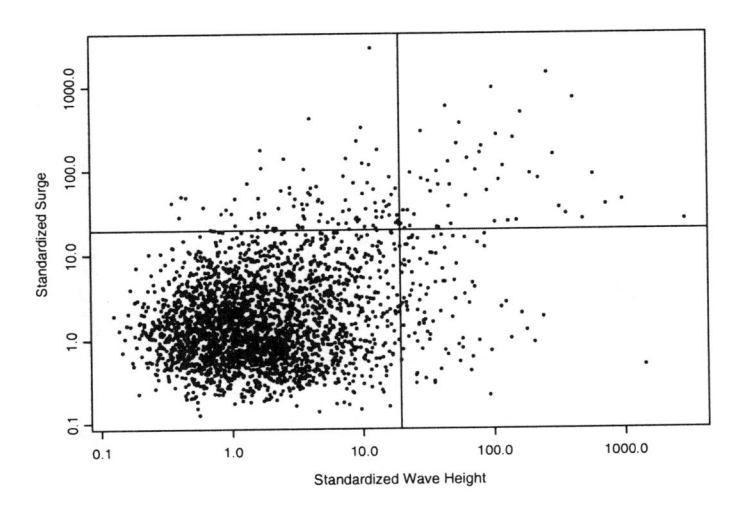

FIGURE 8.6. Plot of wave-surge pairs in Example 1.10 after transformation to Fréchet scale.

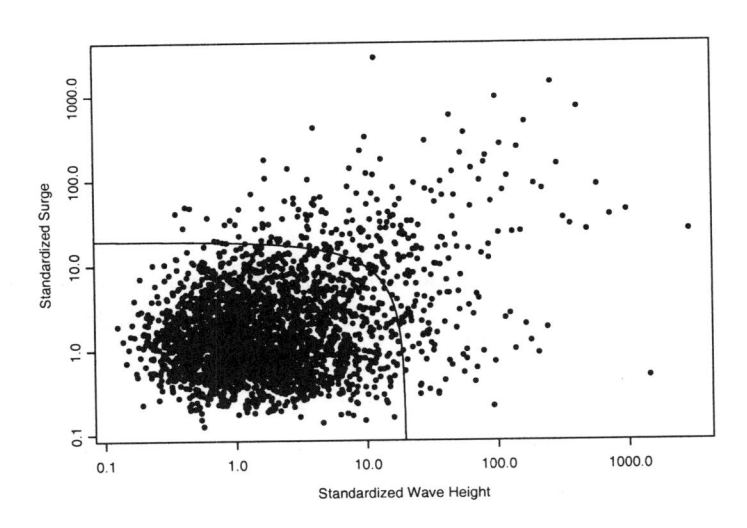

FIGURE 8.7. Plot of wave-surge pairs in Example 1.10 after transformation to Fréchet scale. Threshold shown corresponds to point process model.

160   8. Multivariate Extremes

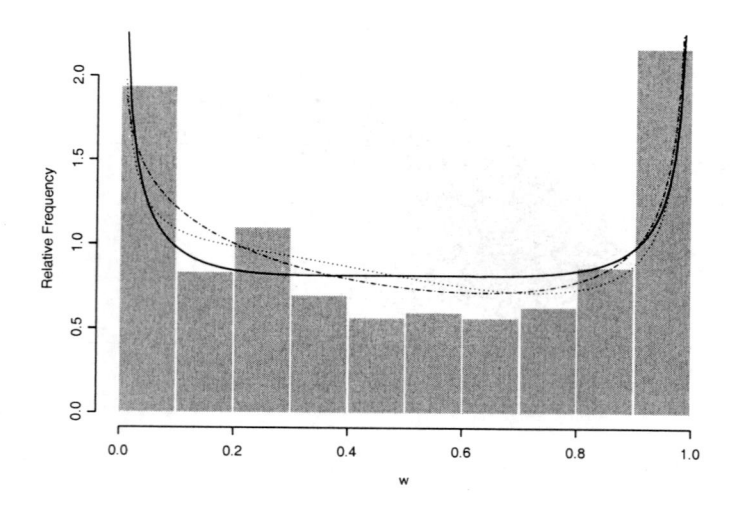

FIGURE 8.8. Histogram of w values in point process analysis of wave-surge data of Example 1.10. Lines show estimates of $h(w)$: logistic model (solid line); bilogistic model (dotted line); Dirichlet model (broken line).

TABLE 8.2. Results of fitting various point process models to the wave-surge data. Values given are maximized log-likelihood (ℓ) and maximum likelihood estimates of α and (where appropriate) β.

Model	ℓ	α	β
Logistic	227.2	0.659	
Bilogistic	230.2	0.704	0.603
Dirichlet	238.2	0.852	0.502

the linearity of the boundary is perturbed, leading to the boundary shown in Fig. 8.7. The region to the right of this boundary is regarded as sufficiently extreme for the point process limit result to provide a valid approximation. A histogram of the observed values of w obtained from (8.24) is shown in Fig. 8.8. The histogram appears flat (though non-zero) for most values of w, but with peaks close to zero and one. This implies that most observations tend to be much greater (on a Fréchet scale) in one variable than the other, though a number of events are large in both components. Maximizing the likelihood (8.28) leads to an estimate of $\hat{\alpha} = 0.659$ for the logistic model, with a standard error of 0.013. A comparison of the fit of this model with the two asymmetric models defined in Section 8.2.1 is given in Table 8.2. Since the logistic model is a subset of the bilogistic model, a formal likelihood ratio test can be used to compare the two. This leads to a deviance test statistic of 6, which is large when compared to a χ_1^2 distribution. Hence, there is evidence of asymmetry in the dependence structure. The likelihood improves further by use of the Dirichlet model. Formal comparison is not possible because the models are no longer nested, but the fact that there is a substantial improvement in likelihood relative to the bilogistic model, which has the same number of parameters, suggests it is a better model. The estimated density $h(w)$ for each of the models is added to the histogram of observed w values in Fig. 8.8. The apparent differences between the models are not great, but it is clear why both of the asymmetric models offer an improvement on the logistic model.

Ignoring the issue of asymmetry, the conclusions from the threshold excess and point process likelihoods based on the logistic model are consistent: dependence is weak but significant. However, the actual estimates of α are different in the two models, even after allowance for sampling error. The differences are due to the different regions on which the model approximations are assumed to be valid. First, the boundaries in Figs. 8.6 and 8.7 are different. More fundamentally, the point process model assumes the validity of the point process limit in the entire region bounded by the threshold boundary and the axes. In particular, it assumes the limit to be reasonable when either of the standardized variables is close to zero, provided the other variable is large. In contrast, the bivariate threshold model assumes accuracy of the limit model only in the joint upper quadrant $R_{1,1}$; information from the other quadrants is censored in the likelihood (8.22). This is achieved at the cost of a large standard error, relative to the point process model, due to the reduction in information that contributes to the likelihood. Choice between the two likelihoods is therefore a familiar bias-variance trade-off.

Closer agreement between models is obtained for the exchange rate data of Example 1.11. As for the Dow Jones Index series, the strong non-stationarity in each of the original exchange rate series can be largely overcome by making a transformation to log-daily returns. Scatterplots of concurrent values of the US/UK and Canadian/UK exchange rates, af-

162   8. Multivariate Extremes

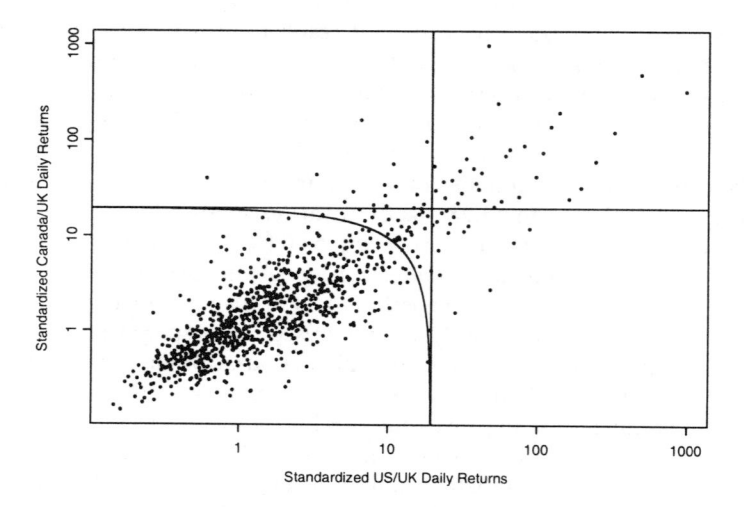

FIGURE 8.9. Plot of log-daily return pairs in Example 1.11 after transformation to Fréchet scale. Thresholds shown correspond to bivariate excess model (solid line) and point process model (broken line).

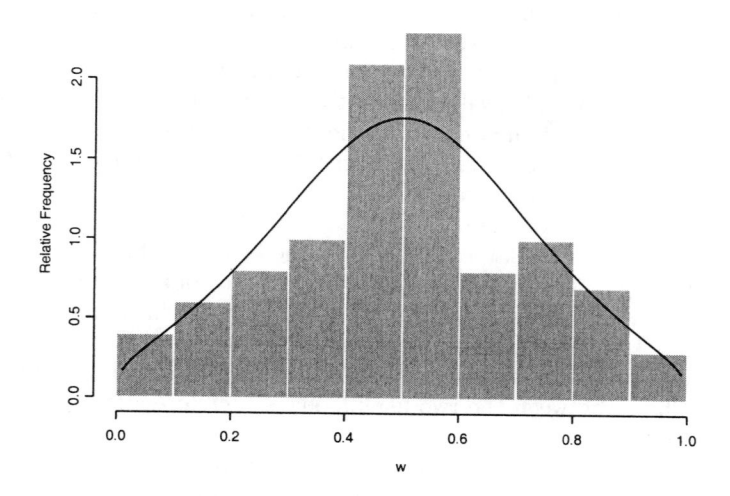

FIGURE 8.10. Histogram of w values in point process analysis of exchange rate data of Example 1.11. Solid line shows $h(w)$ based on fitted logistic model.

ter transformation to a Fréchet scale, are shown in Fig. 8.9. Thresholds for both models are chosen to intersect the axes at the marginal 95% quantiles. The threshold excess model leads to $\hat{\alpha} = 0.464$, with a standard error of 0.039, while the point process model estimate is $\hat{\alpha} = 0.434$, with a standard error of 0.025. The smaller estimate of α for these data confirms the stronger dependence, which seemed apparent from Fig. 8.9. Analyses based on the point process likelihood using both the bilogistic and Dirichlet models leads to negligible improvements in likelihood for these data. So, in contrast with the wave-surge data, there is no evidence for asymmetry in the extremal dependence structure. The estimated logistic model $h(w)$ is compared against a histogram of the w_i values in Fig. 8.10. The unimodality of the histogram suggests a greater tendency for both components of the data to be extreme, while the agreement between model and empirical estimates supports the model choice.

8.4 Asymptotic Independence

When modeling bivariate extremes with either the threshold excess or point process models a particular difficulty can arise. We observed in Section 8.2.1 that a valid limiting distribution in (8.4) is independence:

$$G(x,y) = \exp(-1/x) \times \exp(-1/y), \quad x > 0, \, y > 0.$$

The same applies, therefore, in (8.8). For example, if (X, Y) is a bivariate normal random vector, with any value of the correlation coefficient $\rho < 1$, the limit in (8.8) can be shown to be that of independent variables. On the other hand, especially if ρ is close to 1, observed data are likely to exhibit reasonably strong dependence, even at moderately extreme levels. Hence, models fitted to the data are likely to overestimate dependence on extrapolation.

Suppose, in the first instance, that variables X and Y have a common distribution function F. We define

$$\chi = \lim_{z \to z_+} \Pr\{Y > z \mid X > z\},$$

where z_+ is the end-point of F, so that χ is a limiting measure of the tendency for one variable to be large conditional on the other variable being large. If $\chi = 0$ the variables X and Y are said to be **asymptotically independent**. It is in this situation that the difficulties described above arise. More generally, suppose that F_X and F_Y are the marginal distribution functions of X and Y respectively, and define

$$\chi = \lim_{u \to 1} \Pr\{F_Y(Y) > u \mid F_X(X) > u\}.$$

Defining also, for $0 < u < 1$,

$$\chi(u) = 2 - \frac{\log \Pr\{F_X(X) < u, F_Y(Y) < u\}}{\log \Pr\{F_X(X) < u\}}$$
$$= 2 - \frac{\log \Pr\{F_X(X) < u, F_Y(Y) < u\}}{\log u},$$

it is straightforward to show that

$$\chi = \lim_{u \to 1} \chi(u).$$

It is also easily checked that, for the bivariate extreme value distribution having distribution function $G(x, y) = \exp\{-V(x, y)\}$,

$$\chi(u) = 2 - V(1, 1)$$

uniformly for u. Summarizing, we obtain the following properties for χ:

1. $0 \leq \chi \leq 1$;

2. for the bivariate extreme value distribution, with distribution function $G(x, y) = \exp\{-V(x, y)\}$, $\chi = 2 - V(1, 1)$;

3. for asymptotically independent variables, $\chi = 0$;

4. within the class of asymptotically dependent variables, the value of χ increases with strength of dependence at extreme levels.

From the properties listed above, it is clear that χ provides a simple measure of extremal dependence within the class of asymptotically dependent distributions. It fails, however, to provide any measure of discrimination for asymptotically independent distributions. An alternative measure is required to overcome this deficiency. For $0 < u < 1$, let

$$\bar{\chi}(u) = \frac{2 \log \Pr\{F_X(X) > u\}}{\log \Pr\{F_X(X) > u, F_Y(Y) > u\}} - 1$$
$$= \frac{2 \log(1 - u)}{\log \Pr\{F_X(X) > u, F_Y(Y) > u\}} - 1$$

and

$$\bar{\chi} = \lim_{u \to 1} \bar{\chi}(u).$$

The following properties are easily established:

1. $-1 \leq \bar{\chi} \leq 1$;

2. for asymptotically dependent variables, $\bar{\chi} = 1$;

3. for independent variables, $\bar{\chi} = 0$;

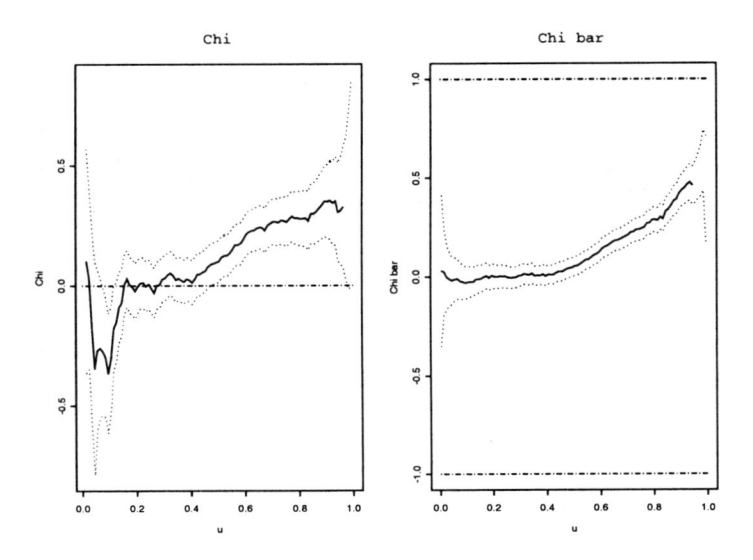

FIGURE 8.11. Empirical estimates of $\chi(u)$ and $\bar{\chi}(u)$ for wave-surge data of Example 1.10. Dotted lines correspond to approximate 95% confidence intervals.

4. for asymptotically independent variables, $\bar{\chi}$ increases with strength of dependence at extreme levels.

It follows that, just as χ provides a measure with which to summarize the strength of dependence within the class of asymptotically dependent variables, so $\bar{\chi}$ provides a corresponding measure within the class of asymptotically independent variables. Taken together, the pair $(\chi, \bar{\chi})$ provides a summary of extremal dependence for an arbitrary random vector. If $\bar{\chi} = 1$, the variables are asymptotically dependent, and the value of χ summarizes the strength of extremal dependence; if $\bar{\chi} < 1$, then $\chi = 0$, the variables are asymptotically independent, and the value of $\bar{\chi}$ is more appropriate as a measure of the strength of extremal dependence.

Replacing probabilities with observed proportions enables empirical estimates of $\chi(u)$ and $\bar{\chi}(u)$ to be calculated and used as a means of model assessment. In particular, estimates can be plotted as functions of u to ascertain the limiting behavior as $u \to 1$. For componentwise block maxima models there are usually insufficient data to overcome the large sampling variation in the empirical estimates. For the threshold and point process models, however, the technique can be useful in distinguishing between asymptotic dependence and asymptotic independence, for determining suitable thresholds, and for validating the choice of a particular model for V.

As an illustration, the plots of empirical estimates of $\chi(u)$ and $\bar{\chi}(u)$, together with approximate 95% confidence intervals, are shown for the wave-surge data of Example 1.10 in Fig. 8.11, and for the log-daily return

166   8. Multivariate Extremes

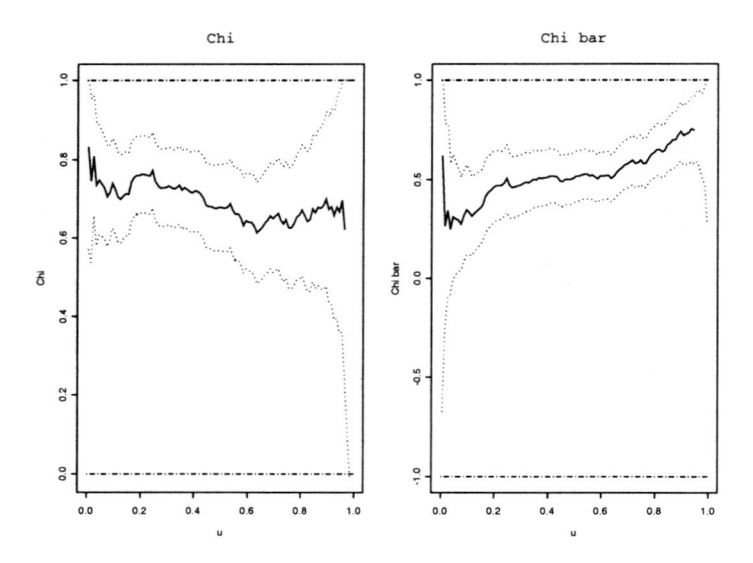

FIGURE 8.12. Empirical estimates of $\chi(u)$ and $\bar{\chi}(u)$ for log-daily return pairs of Example 1.11. Dotted lines correspond to approximate 95% confidence intervals.

exchange rate data of Example 1.11 in Fig. 8.12. Interpretation is not completely straightforward because of the large variance of the estimators, but both sets of figures seem consistent with the possibility that $\bar{\chi}(u) \to 1$ as $u \to 1$. In the respective examples, $\chi(u)$ converges to values of around 0.3 and 0.65. These observations lend support to the use of asymptotically dependent models above sufficiently high thresholds. Moreover, stability of $\chi(u)$ in both examples seems plausible for $u \geq 0.95$, suggesting that the use of 95% marginal quantiles as thresholds is reasonable. Finally, since

$$\chi = 2 - V(1,1) = 2 - 2^\alpha \qquad (8.29)$$

for the logistic model, we can obtain the maximum likelihood estimate of χ by substitution of the maximum likelihood estimate of α into (8.29). For the wave-surge and exchange rate threshold excess model analyses we obtain $\hat{\chi} = 0.309$ and $\hat{\chi} = 0.621$ respectively. Each value is consistent with the apparent stable-levels of $\bar{\chi}(u)$ in Figs. 8.11 and 8.12 respectively, providing additional evidence of goodness-of-fit.

In situations where diagnostic checks suggest data to be asymptotically independent, modeling with the classical families of bivariate extreme value distributions and their threshold equivalents is likely to lead to misleading results. In this case, under mild assumptions, limit results can be obtained for the rate of convergence to independence. In turn, these results can be used to construct appropriate families of models. The articles by Ledford & Tawn referred to in the next section cover this issue in some depth.

8.5 Further Reading

General aspects of the difficulties in working with multivariate distributions, including the problem of defining what is meant by a multivariate extreme event, are discussed by Barnett (1976).

The characterization of multivariate extreme value distributions based on point process arguments was first developed by de Haan & Resnick (1977). Pickands (1981) gives an equivalent representation, while de Haan (1985a) includes discussion on inferential aspects of the model. A detailed, if technical, development of the fundamental representations is given in Chapter 5 of Resnick (1987). The development of sub-families of extreme value models is somewhat older: see Gumbel (1960) and Tiago de Oliveira (1984a) for example.

Elementary approaches to obtaining summary measures of dependence between extremes of different variables have been proposed in a variety of contexts: references include Buishand (1984, 1991) and Dales & Reed (1988).

Statistical modeling with multivariate extreme value distributions is comparatively recent and remains an area of rapid development. Tawn (1988a) developed parametric models and inferential techniques for the componentwise block maximum model. Coles & Tawn (1991) and Joe et al. (1992) independently proposed modeling directly with the point process characterization; Coles & Tawn (1994) discuss many of the practical issues involved with such an approach. Coles & Tawn (1991) and Joe et al. (1992) also include techniques for developing families of multivariate extreme value models; other techniques and models are discussed by Joe (1989, 1994) and Tawn (1990). Reviews of the statistical aspects of multivariate extreme value modeling are given by Smith (1994) and Tawn (1994). Bruun & Tawn (1998) provide a detailed comparison of multivariate and structure variable methods.

The use of multivariate extreme value techniques for financial applications has also received considerable attention in recent years. For example, Hüsler (1996) is one of several articles in a special volume under the heading 'Multivariate extreme value estimation with applications to economics and finance'.

Nonparametric estimation of multivariate extreme value models is also natural because of the functional representation in (8.5). Smith et al. (1990), for example, compared parametric and nonparametric techniques based on kernel smoothing for modeling componentwise block maxima. There have also been many nonparametric techniques proposed on the basis of threshold models: Deheuvels & Tiago de Oliveira (1989), Einmahl et al. (1993, 1997), Capéraà et al. (1997) and Hall & Tajvidi (2000a) for example.

The original proof of asymptotic independence of the bivariate normal family is due to Sibuya (1960). The more recent attention given to the statistical properties of asymptotically independent distributions is largely a result of a series of articles by Jonathan Tawn and Anthony Ledford: Ledford & Tawn (1996), Ledford & Tawn (1997) and Ledford & Tawn (1998). Coles et al. (1999) give an elementary synthesis of this theory.

Extensions of the characterizations of multivariate extremes to stationary processes have also been developed: Hsing (1989), for example.

9
Further Topics

9.1 Bayesian Inference

9.1.1 General Theory

In Chapter 3 we discussed a number of different techniques for parameter estimation in extreme value models and argued that likelihood-based methods are preferable. Subsequently, all our analyses have adopted the procedure of maximum likelihood. But this is not the only way to draw inferences from the likelihood function, and Bayesian techniques offer an alternative that is often preferable.

The general set-up for a Bayesian analysis is the following. As in Chapter 2, we assume data $x = (x_1, \ldots, x_n)$ to be realizations of a random variable whose density falls within a parametric family $\mathcal{F} = \{f(x; \theta) : \theta \in \Theta\}$. However, we now assume it is possible to formulate beliefs about θ, without reference to the data, that can be expressed as a probability distribution. For example, if we are sure that $0 \leq \theta \leq 1$, but that any value in that range is equally likely, our beliefs could be expressed by the probability distribution $\theta \sim \mathrm{U}(0, 1)$. On the other hand, if θ is real-valued and we believe that θ is likely to be small in magnitude rather than large, a distribution of the form $\theta \sim \mathrm{N}(0, 100)$ may be more appropriate. A distribution on the parameter θ, made without reference to the data, is termed a **prior distribution**. Specification of a prior distribution represents a substantial departure from the inferential framework we discussed in Chapter 2, in which parameters were implicitly assumed to be constant. Admittedly unknown, but nevertheless constant. In the Bayesian setting, parameters are treated as random variables, and the prior distribution consists of the parameter distribution prior to the inclusion of additional information provided by data. This specification of information in the form of a prior distribution is regarded alternately as the greatest strength and the main pitfall of Bayesian inference. Protagonists argue that the prior distribution enables the statistician to supplement the information provided by data, which is often very limited, with other sources of relevant information. In contrast, antagonists contend that, since different analysts would specify different priors, all conclusions become meaninglessly subjective.

Postponing, for the moment, the arguments for and against the methodology, let $f(\theta)$ denote the density of the prior distribution for θ.[1] With a slight abuse of notation in which f is used generically to denote an arbitrary density function, we can also write the likelihood for θ as $f(x \mid \theta)$. For example, if the x_i are independent, then

$$f(x \mid \theta) = \prod_{i=1}^{n} f(x_i; \theta).$$

Bayes' Theorem states

$$f(\theta \mid x) = \frac{f(\theta) f(x \mid \theta)}{\int_\Theta f(\theta) f(x \mid \theta) d\theta}. \tag{9.1}$$

In the context of probability theory, Bayes' Theorem is unchallengeable: it is an immediate consequence of the axioms of probability and the definition of conditional probability. In the context of statistical analysis, its use is revolutionary. It provides the machinery for converting an initial set of beliefs about θ, as represented by the prior distribution $f(\theta)$, into a **posterior distribution**, $f(\theta \mid x)$, that includes the additional information provided by the data x. Furthermore, Bayes' Theorem leads to an inference that comprises a complete distribution. This means that the accuracy of an inference can be summarized, for example, by the variance of the posterior distribution, without the need to resort to asymptotic theory. Decision-theoretic considerations also lead to non-arbitrary choices of point estimators of θ. For example, the posterior mean is found to be the estimate that minimizes expected quadratic loss. This contrasts with the *ad hoc*, albeit intuitive, rationale for maximum likelihood.

Prediction is also neatly handled within a Bayesian setting. If z denotes a future observation having probability density function $f(z \mid \theta)$, and $f(\theta \mid x)$ denotes the posterior distribution of θ on the basis of observed data x, then

$$f(z \mid x) = \int_\Theta f(z \mid \theta) f(\theta \mid x) d\theta \tag{9.2}$$

---

[1]The case in which θ is defined on a discrete space follows in the same way, with obvious adjustments to terminology.

is the **predictive density** of z given x. Compared with other approaches to prediction, the predictive density has the advantage that it reflects uncertainty in the model – the $f(\theta \mid x)$ term – and uncertainty due to the variability in future observations – the $f(z \mid \theta)$ term.

So, if you accept the price of having to specify a prior distribution, which many regard as an advantage in itself, there are strong pragmatic reasons to prefer a Bayesian analysis. The main obstacle to the widespread adoption of Bayesian techniques – apart from philosophical objections to the subjectivity induced by the use of prior distributions – is the difficulty of computation: posterior inference usually requires integration in (9.1). Judicious choice of prior families can, for certain likelihood models, avoid the necessity to calculate the normalizing integral in (9.1), but this simplification is the exception rather than the rule. For complex models, where θ may be a high-dimensional vector of parameters, computation of the denominator in (9.1) can be problematic, even using sophisticated numerical integration techniques. This difficulty has recently been tackled by the development of simulation-based techniques. One technique in particular, Markov chain Monte Carlo (MCMC), has popularized the use of Bayesian techniques to the extent that they are now standard in many areas of application.

The idea is simple: to produce simulated values from the posterior distribution in (9.1). If this could be done exactly, the simulated sample could be used to obtain estimates of the posterior distribution itself. For example, the mean of the simulated values would give an estimate of the posterior mean; a histogram of the simulated values would give an estimate of the posterior density; and so on. The difficulty is knowing how to simulate from $f(\theta \mid x)$, and usually this is not achievable. The technique of MCMC is to simulate a sequence $\theta_1, \theta_2, \ldots$ in the following way: set an initial value θ_1, and specify an *arbitrary* probability rule $q(\theta_{i+1} \mid \theta_i)$ for iterative simulation of successive values. Possibilities include $(\theta_{i+1} \mid \theta_i) \sim N(\theta_i, 1)$ or $(\theta_{i+1} \mid \theta_i) \sim \text{Gamma}(1,1)$.[2] This procedure generates a first-order Markov chain[3] since, given θ_i, the stochastic properties of θ_{i+1} are independent of the earlier history $\theta_1, \ldots, \theta_{i-1}$. But, in this way, the evolution of the θ_i depends on the arbitrary q, rather than the target density given in (9.1). The trick, at each step in the sequence, is to use the probability rule $q(\cdot \mid \theta_i)$ to generate a proposal value θ^* for θ_{i+1}, but to reject this proposal in favor of θ_i with a specified probability. Specifically, letting

$$\alpha_i = \min\left\{1, \frac{f(x \mid \theta^*)f(\theta^*)q(\theta_i \mid \theta^*)}{f(x \mid \theta_i)f(\theta_i)q(\theta^* \mid \theta_i)}\right\}, \qquad (9.3)$$

---

[2] In the second of these examples, the distribution of θ_{i+1} does not depend on θ_i. This is said to be an independence sampler.

[3] See Section 2.4.2.

we set

$$\theta_{i+1} = \begin{cases} \theta^* & \text{with probability } \alpha_i, \\ \theta_i & \text{with probability } 1 - \alpha_i. \end{cases} \qquad (9.4)$$

By construction, the generated sequence is still a Markov chain, but now having a stationary distribution which, under simple regularity assumptions, can be shown to be the target distribution (9.1). This implies that, for a large enough value of k, the sequence $\theta_{k+1}, \theta_{k+2}, \ldots$ is approximately stationary, with marginal distribution given by (9.1). This sequence can therefore be used in a similar way to a sequence of independent values to estimate features such as the posterior mean. It's almost like magic: regardless of the choice of q,[4] the rejection steps implied by (9.4) ensure that the simulated values have, in a limiting sense, the desired marginal distribution. In reality, there is a lot more to the story, since choosing q so as to ensure a short settling-in period, and to generate low dependence in the sequence, can be difficult to arrange. Nonetheless, MCMC procedures create the opportunity to explore the use of Bayesian techniques in application areas that were previously thought of as impenetrable due to the computations implied by (9.1).

9.1.2 Bayesian Inference of Extremes

There are a number of reasons why a Bayesian analysis of extreme value data might be desirable. First and foremost, owing to scarcity of data, the facility to include other sources of information through a prior distribution has obvious appeal. Second, as we have discussed, the output of a Bayesian analysis – the posterior distribution – provides a more complete inference than the corresponding maximum likelihood analysis. In particular, since the objective of an extreme value analysis is usually an estimate of the probability of future events reaching extreme levels, expression through predictive distributions is natural. For example, a suitable model for the annual maximum Z of a process is $Z \sim \text{GEV}(\mu, \sigma, \xi)$. Estimation of $\theta = (\mu, \sigma, \xi)$ could be made on the basis of previous daily observations $x = (x_1, \ldots, x_n)$ using, for example, the point process model of Chapter 7. If this is done via a Bayesian analysis, the result is a posterior distribution $f(\theta \mid x)$. Then, by (9.2),

$$\Pr\{Z \leq z \mid x_1, \ldots, x_n\} = \int_\Theta \Pr\{Z \leq z \mid \theta\} f(\theta \mid x) d\theta. \qquad (9.5)$$

Consequently, (9.5) gives the distribution of a future annual maximum of the process that allows both for parameter uncertainty and randomness in

---

[4]Subject to some regularity.

future observations. Solving

$$\Pr\{Z \leq z \mid x_1, \ldots, x_n\} = 1 - 1/m \qquad (9.6)$$

therefore gives an analog of the m-year return level that incorporates uncertainty due to model estimation. Whilst (9.5) may seem intractable, it is easily approximated if the posterior distribution has itself been estimated by simulation, using for example MCMC. After deletion of the values generated in the settling-in period, the procedure leads to a sample $\theta_1, \ldots, \theta_s$ that may be regarded as observations from the stationary distribution $f(\theta \mid x)$. Hence, by (9.5),

$$\Pr\{Z \leq z \mid x_1, \ldots, x_n\} \approx \frac{1}{s} \sum_{i=1}^{s} \Pr\{Z \leq z \mid \theta_i\}, \qquad (9.7)$$

and solution of (9.6) is straightforward using a standard numerical solver. A third reason for favoring a Bayesian analysis is that it is not dependent on the regularity assumptions required by the asymptotic theory of maximum likelihood. In particular, in the unusual situation where $\xi < -0.5$ and the classical theory of maximum likelihood breaks down,[5] Bayesian inference provides a viable alternative.

All of these issues are discussed in detail by Coles & Tawn (1996a). They argue that prior elicitation in an extreme value analysis is most reasonably achieved in terms of extreme quantiles of a process, rather than the extreme value model parameters themselves. Subject to self-consistency, a prior distribution on a set of three quantiles can always be transformed to a prior distribution on (μ, σ, ξ). Standard MCMC algorithms can then be applied to obtain realizations from the corresponding posterior distribution which, in turn, can be used to estimate the predictive distribution of, say, the annual maximum distribution through (9.7).

9.1.3 Example: Port Pirie Annual Maximum Sea-levels

To illustrate the methodology, we give a naive Bayesian analysis of the Port Pirie annual maximum sea-level data of Example 1.1. We use the word naive here with two different meanings: first, because we have no external information with which to formulate a prior distribution; second, because we choose an arbitrary configuration of the MCMC algorithm that ensures simplicity of programming, with little attempt to guarantee that the generated chain has good properties.

Specifying a prior distribution is a necessary component of any Bayesian analysis, even if there is no information with which to do so. In such situations it is usual to use priors that have very high variance – or equivalently,

---

[5] See Section 3.3.1.

are near-flat – reflecting the absence of genuine prior information. There is considerable literature on this issue, but in practical terms, analyses are not usually sensitive to choices of prior distribution that have a sufficiently large variance. In any given problem, this aspect can be explored through a sensitivity analysis.

The likelihood model for the Port Pirie analysis is

$$Z_i \sim \text{GEV}(\mu, \sigma, \xi), \quad i = 1, \ldots, 65, \tag{9.8}$$

where Z_i denotes the annual maximum sea-level in the year indexed by i. Setting $\phi = \log \sigma$, we might choose a prior density function

$$f(\mu, \phi, \xi) = f_\mu(\mu) f_\phi(\phi) f_\xi(\xi), \tag{9.9}$$

where $f_\mu(\cdot)$, $f_\phi(\cdot)$ and $f_\xi(\cdot)$ are normal density functions with mean zero and variances v_μ, v_ϕ and v_ξ respectively. The reason for working with ϕ is that it is an easier parameterization with which to respect the positivity on σ. The prior density (9.9) then corresponds to a specification of prior independence in the parameters μ, ϕ and ξ, which can be made to be near-flat by choosing the variance parameters sufficiently large. The choice of normal densities is arbitrary. For this analysis, we chose $v_\mu = v_\phi = 10^4$ and $v_\xi = 100$. This completes the model specification.

For the inference, it is necessary to choose an MCMC algorithm. There is almost unbounded latitude here. For illustration, we adopt a variant on the scheme described in Section 9.1.1, in which steps (9.3) and (9.4) are applied sequentially to each of the individual components of the vector (μ, ϕ, ξ). In other words, (9.3) and (9.4) are applied exactly, but where q is replaced in turn by transition densities q_μ, q_ϕ and q_ξ, each being a function of its own argument only. One simple choice is to specify densities corresponding to random walks in the three component directions:

$$\begin{aligned} \mu^* &= \mu + \epsilon_\mu, \\ \phi^* &= \phi + \epsilon_\phi, \\ \xi^* &= \xi + \epsilon_\xi, \end{aligned}$$

where $\epsilon_\mu, \epsilon_\phi$ and ϵ_ξ are normally distributed variables, with zero means and variances w_μ, w_ϕ and w_ξ respectively. Unlike the prior specification, the choice of algorithm and its tuning parameters – w_μ, w_ϕ and w_ξ for our algorithm – does not affect the model. It does, however, affect the efficiency of the algorithm. After a little trial-and-error, the choices $w_\mu = 0.0004$, $w_\phi = 0.01$ and $w_\xi = 0.01$ were found to work reasonably well in this example.

Initializing with $(\mu, \phi, \xi) = (5, 0, 0.1)$, the values generated by 1000 iterations of the chain are plotted in Fig. 9.1. The settling-in period seems to take around 400 iterations; thereafter, the stochastic variations in the

9.1 Bayesian Inference   175

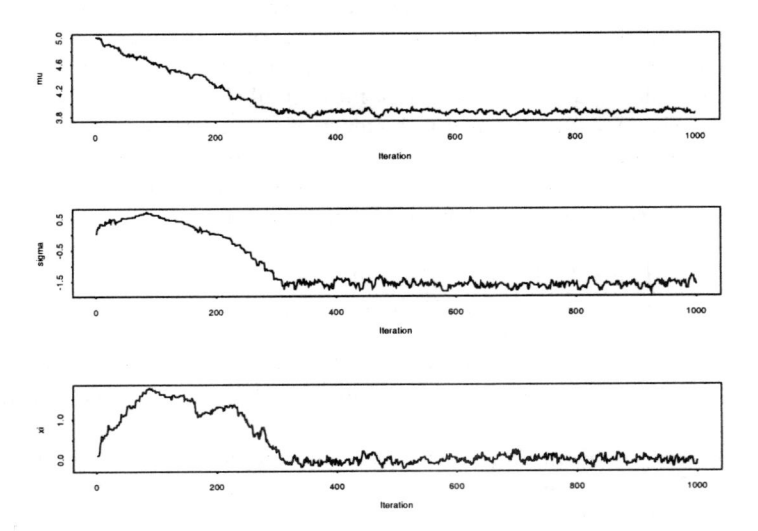

FIGURE 9.1. MCMC realizations of GEV parameters in a Bayesian analysis of the Port Pirie annual maximum sea-levels. Top panel: μ; middle panel: σ; bottom panel: ξ.

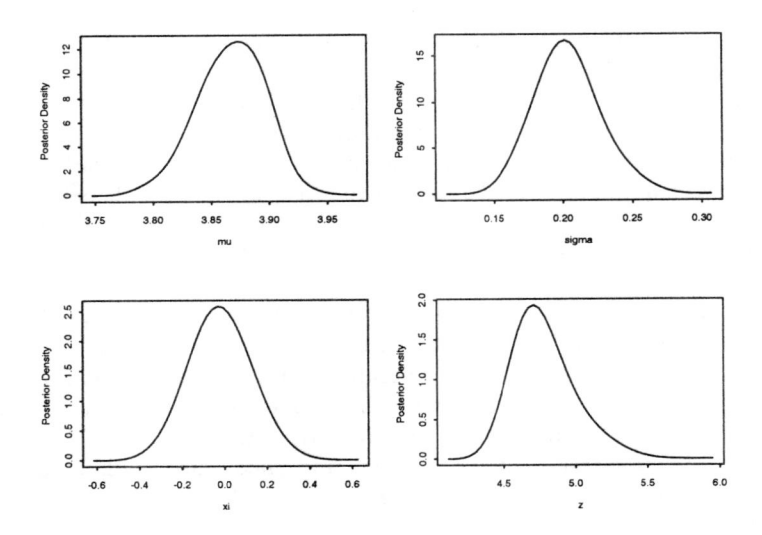

FIGURE 9.2. Estimated posterior densities of GEV parameters and 100-year return level in a Bayesian analysis of Port Pirie annual maximum sea-levels. Top left: μ; top right: σ; bottom left: ξ; bottom right: $z_{0.01}$.

chain seem reasonably homogeneous.[6] If we accept this, after deleting the first 400 simulations, the remaining 600 simulated values can be treated as dependent realizations whose marginal distribution is the target posterior. For comparison with earlier analyses, it is convenient to transform back to the usual σ scale, by setting $\sigma_i = \exp \phi_i$ for each of the simulated ϕ_i values. In a similar way, having obtained a sequence of simulated values (μ_i, σ_i, ξ_i) from the target distribution, the components may be transformed to obtain simulated values from specified functions of these parameters. For example, the $1/p$-year return level was defined in Chapter 3 as

$$z_p = \begin{cases} \mu - \frac{\sigma}{\xi}\left[1 - \{-\log(1-p)\}^{-\xi}\right], & \text{for } \xi \neq 0, \\ \mu - \sigma \log\{-\log(1-p)\}, & \text{for } \xi = 0. \end{cases}$$

Applying this transformation to each of the vectors (μ_i, σ_i, ξ_i) leads to a sample from the corresponding posterior distribution of the $1/p$ year return level.

For the analysis of the Port Pirie data, the sample means and standard deviations (in parentheses) of the simulated values of the model parameters and the 100-year return level are

$\hat{\mu} = 3.87$ (0.03), $\hat{\sigma} = 0.20$ (0.02), $\hat{\xi} = -0.020$ (0.091), $\hat{z}_{0.01} = 4.78$ (0.19).

Since the simulated values are treated as observations from the Markov chain once it has reached equilibrium, these represent calculations of the posterior mean and standard deviation respectively of each of the marginal components. Looking back to Section 3.4.1, the results are similar to, and certainly consistent with, the corresponding estimates based on the maximum likelihood analysis. Given the uninformativeness of the prior specification made, this degree of self-consistency is reassuring. The main advantage of the Bayesian inference in this case is the ease with which the simulated data can be used to give a more complete summary of the analysis. For example, posterior density estimates of the parameters and $z_{0.01}$ are shown in Fig. 9.2.

Using the method discussed in Section 9.1.2, a plot of the predictive distribution of a future annual maximum is shown in Fig. 9.3 on the usual return period scale. The values are greater than the corresponding return level estimates based on a maximum likelihood analysis because of the implicit allowance for uncertainty in parameter estimation.

In summary, the results of the Bayesian and maximum likelihood analyses are mutually consistent, while the Bayesian analysis facilitates an easy transformation across scales that does not depend on asymptotic properties of the likelihood function. Moreover, uncertainty in prediction, due to

---

[6]See Gilks et al. (1996) for a discussion of formal diagnostic procedures for chain convergence.

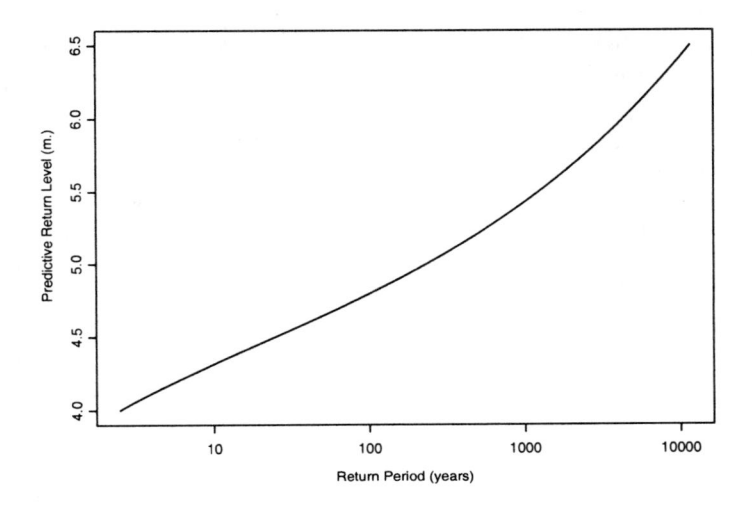

FIGURE 9.3. Predictive return levels z_p against $1/p$, where $\Pr\{Z \leq z_p \mid \boldsymbol{x}\} = 1 - 1/p$, in a Bayesian analysis of Port Pirie annual maximum sea-level series.

parameter uncertainty, is more naturally expressed in the Bayesian framework. The computations for the Bayesian analysis are straightforward and fast – this simple example ran at virtually the same speed as the maximum likelihood analysis. Modifications to handle non-stationarity and other perturbations from the standard model assumptions can also be included. Similarly, although we have illustrated the method using the GEV sample maxima model, the basic strategy applies equally well for any of the other extreme value models we have introduced. Together with the fact that genuine external information can additionally be incorporated into the inference through the prior distribution, the Bayesian framework offers substantial advantages for the analysis of extreme values.

9.2 Extremes of Markov Chains

We argued in Section 5.3.2 that a pragmatic way of modeling extremes of a stationary process is to decluster the data and then apply the standard threshold excess model to the cluster maxima only. This is justified by the asymptotic theory which leads to the generalized Pareto distribution as being the limiting distribution of threshold excesses. The declustering is an ad hoc device to circumvent the difficulty that the joint distribution of successive threshold excesses is unspecified by the general theory. But there are disadvantages to this approach: cluster identification is often arbitrary; information on extremes is discarded; and the opportunity for modeling within-cluster behavior is lost. This latter point can be especially important in some applications if, for example, the cumulative effect of extreme values is critical.

Because the general results are not more prescriptive, the only way to avoid the declustering method that is supported by asymptotic theory is to make stronger assumptions about the process under study. The simplest assumption that might be made, other than independence, is that the series $X_1, X_2, \ldots$ forms a stationary first-order Markov chain. Smith et al. (1997) proposed a general framework for modeling extremes of such series. A brief summary follows.

The stochastic properties of a stationary first-order Markov chain are completely determined by the distribution of successive pairs. This is because the joint density factorizes as

$$f(x_1, \ldots, x_n) = f(x_1) \times f(x_2 \mid x_1) \times f(x_3 \mid x_2) \times \cdots \times f(x_n \mid x_{n-1})$$

due to the Markov property. Given a model $f(x_i, x_{i+1}; \theta)$, it follows that the likelihood for θ is

$$L(\theta) = f(x_1) \prod_{i=1}^{n-1} f(x_{i+1} \mid x_i; \theta) = f(x_1) \frac{\prod_{i=1}^{n-1} f(x_i, x_{i+1}; \theta)}{\prod_{i=1}^{n-1} f(x_i; \theta)}.$$

Adopting the asymptotic arguments of Chapters 4 and 8, approximate models for both $f(x_i; \theta)$ and $f(x_i, x_{i+1}; \theta)$ are available on regions of the form (u, ∞) and $(u, \infty) \times (u, \infty)$ respectively, from (4.11) and (8.5). Below the chosen thresholds, the model is unspecified and it is necessary to censor the likelihood components as in Section 8.3.1. Once estimated, simulation of clusters from the fitted model can be used to estimate other characteristics of the process such as the extremal index. An analytical expression for the extremal index of a first-order Markov chain is given by Smith (1992), but the estimation of other extremal features of the series requires the more general modeling methodology of Smith et al. (1997).

Though Markov chains are a simplification of the types of dependence often encountered in real datasets, they provide a much more plausible set of assumptions than independence. Consequently, the generalization of modeling procedures for extremes of independent series to that of first-order Markov chains greatly expands the applicability of extreme value techniques to the modeling of extremes of genuine data processes. The generalization to higher-order Markov chains is also straightforward, apart from the difficulties of increased dimensionality discussed in Chapter 8.

9.3 Spatial Extremes

In Chapter 8 we argued that one reason for considering a multivariate analysis of extremes would be if the joint probability of extreme events at a number of different locations were of interest. This argument generalizes in the following way. Consider, for example, a continuous stretch of coastline, with locations indexed by $r \in R = [0, 1]$, and let $X(r)$ denote the sea-level at location r. Assuming a sea-wall to have a constant height of u along the coastline, the probability of an exceedance of the sea-wall at any location is

$$1 - \Pr\{X(r) < u \ \forall r \in R\}. \tag{9.10}$$

Other quantities may also be of interest: for example, with $a_+ = \max\{0, a\}$,

$$\int_R \{X(r) - u\}_+ dr \tag{9.11}$$

is the total volume of water exceeding the sea-wall. Calculation of either (9.10) or (9.11) requires a specification of the joint probability of extreme events across the whole index space R, or, in other words, the extremal properties of the sea-level regarded as a continuous spatial process.

The argument generalizes further to spatial problems in which the underlying space is two-dimensional. For example, letting R be an index space for the catchment region in a hydrological analysis, and denoting by $X(r)$ the daily rainfall at location $r \in R$, calculations of the type

$$1 - \Pr\{X(r) < u(r) \ \forall r \in R\},$$

for a specified function $u(r)$, can be used to evaluate the probability of flood levels in at least one location in the region.

Two proposals have been made for modeling spatial extremes, one based on a continuous version of the extremal types theorem, the other related to standard methodology for spatial statistics. Both approaches are computationally intensive and implementations have so far been largely exploratory. It remains to be seen if the models can be developed for routine use.

9.3.1 Max-stable Processes

Max-stable processes are a continuous analog of max-stable random variables. As in the multivariate case, it is convenient to give definitions with reference to a standard Fréchet marginal distribution.

Definition 9.1 Let $X(r)$ be a random process on an index space R, with standard Fréchet margins, and let $X_1(r), X_2(r), \ldots$ be independent replications of the $X(r)$ process. For $n = 1, 2, \ldots$, let $Z_n(r)$ be such that, for each $r \in R$,

$$Z_n(r) = \max_{i=1,\ldots,n} \{X_i(r)\}. \tag{9.12}$$

Then, $X(r)$ is said to be a **max-stable process** if, for each $n = 1, 2, \ldots$, it is identical in distribution to $n^{-1} Z_n(r)$. △

The definition of $Z_n(r)$ in (9.12) is analogous to the definition of componentwise block maxima on discrete spaces. Similarly, the property of max-stability for random processes is a generalization of max-stable random variables: up to scaling, the distribution of a max-stable process is invariant to the operation of taking pointwise maxima.

The correspondence between max-stable variables and max-stable processes extends to a continuous version of the extremal types theorem.

Theorem 9.1 Let $X(r)$ be a random process with standard Fréchet margins on an index space R, and let

$$Z_n^*(r) = \max_{i=1,\ldots,n} \{X_i(r)/n\}.$$

Then, if

$$Z_n^*(r) \xrightarrow{d} Z(r)$$

as $n \to \infty$, where $Z(r)$ is a well-defined process, $Z(r)$ is a max-stable process. □

By Theorem 9.1, max-stable processes are the limits of pointwise maxima processes in the same way that the GEV family is the limit distribution of block maxima, and the bivariate extreme value family is the limit distribution of componentwise block maxima. This analogy suggests the use of the limit family as an approximation to $Z_n^*(r)$ in a manner that is now familiar. But this requires a characterization of the limit family. One characterization, which is a continuous version of the point process representation for multivariate extremes, is given by the following spectral representation due to de Haan (1985b).

Theorem 9.2 Let $\{(u_1, s_1), (u_2, s_2), \ldots\}$ be the points of a Poisson process on a space $(0, \infty) \times S$, with intensity density function

$$\lambda(du, ds) = \frac{du}{u^2} \times \nu(ds)$$

for a positive intensity function ν on S. Also, let f be a function on $R \times S$ such that

$$\int_S f(r, s)\nu(ds) = 1, \quad \forall \, r \in R. \tag{9.13}$$

Then setting

$$Z(r) = \max_{i=1,2,\ldots} \{u_i f(r, s_i)\},$$

$Z(r)$ is a max-stable process. Moreover, every max-stable process on R can be represented in this way for suitable choices of S, ν and f. □

It is easy from this representation to show that, for any subset $R_0 \subset R$,

$$\Pr\{X(r) \leq u(r) \ \forall \ r \in R_0\} = \exp\left\{-\int_S \max_{r \in R_0} \left(\frac{f(r,s)}{u(r)}\right) \nu(ds)\right\},$$

which is an infinite-dimensional version of the limit distribution for bivariate componentwise maxima given by (8.5).

Smith (1991b) gave the following physical interpretation to the characterization in Theorem 9.2.

- The space S is to be interpreted as a space of 'storm types', for example 'storm locations'.

- The function ν determines the relative frequency of different storm types.

- The intensity function λ determines the joint intensity of storm types and severity, which are assumed to be mutually independent.

- The function $f(r,s)$ is interpreted as a 'storm profile function', determining the relative strength of a storm of type s observed at r, so that $u_i f(r, s_i)$ is the severity of the ith storm measured at r.

- Finally, $Z(r)$ is obtained by maximizing storm severity over all storms at each location r.

Smith (1991b) exploited this interpretation to build a class of max-stable processes having a simple physical interpretation. In his model, $S = R$, with S interpreted as a space of storm centers, and $\nu(ds) = ds$, corresponding to a uniform spread of storm centers. Finally, any family of probability density functions $f(\cdot, s)$, where s is a parameter of f, provides a model for $f(r,s)$ that satisfies (9.13). In particular, setting $f(r,s) = \phi(r-s)$, where $\phi(\cdot)$ is the standard normal density function, leads to a model for which a number of analytical properties can be evaluated. These properties, in turn, enable a method of inference based on a weighted least-squares smoothing of empirical and model-based estimates of pairwise dependence.

9.3.2 Latent Spatial Process Models

An alternative approach for specifying extreme value models over continuous spaces is by the use of latent spatial processes. For example, suppose we make observations of annual maxima, $X(r_i)$, at a set of locations $r_1, \ldots, r_k \in R$. A possible latent process model is

$$X(r_i) \mid (\mu_1, \ldots, \mu_k, \sigma, \xi) \sim \text{GEV}(\mu_i, \sigma, \xi) \qquad (9.14)$$

independently for $r_1, \ldots, r_k$, where $\mu_1, \ldots, \mu_k$ are the realizations of a smoothly varying random process $\mu(r)$ observed at $r = r_1, \ldots, r_k$ respectively. Because $\mu(r)$ varies smoothly, nearby values of the $\mu(r_i)$ are more likely to be similar than distant values. Hence, values of $X(r)$ are more likely to be similar at nearby locations. Thus, dependence is induced, as a consequence of the smoothness in the hidden $\mu(r)$ process.

Compared with max-stable processes, model specification is easier using latent processes and, although the computational burden is substantial, analyses with quite large numbers of locations are still manageable. A limitation is that strong dependence cannot be induced in this way, and the technique is likely to have greater utility as a method for inferring smooth variations in GEV model parameters, rather than as a serious proposition for modeling spatial dependence.

9.4 Further Reading

A general overview of the use of Bayesian techniques can be found in Casella & Berger (2001) or O'Hagan (1994). Specific details on MCMC modeling are given by Gilks et al. (1996), though the area is rapidly developing. While there is a large literature on Bayesian inference for extreme value models, much of it is restricted to special cases and sub-models. In the context of modeling with the complete GEV family, the earliest reference seems to be Smith & Naylor (1987). Coles & Powell (1996) give a more general review and also discuss contemporary modeling ideas based on Markov chain Monte Carlo techniques. Using this methodology, Coles & Tawn (1996a) provide a case study that demonstrates the utility of expert information for extreme value modeling. Walshaw (2000) extends these simple ideas to hidden mixture models. An interestind discussion of the relative merits of Bayesian and frequentist estimates of predictive quantities for extremes is given by Smith (1999).

Theoretical properties of extremes of Markov chains are given by Smith (1992) and Perfekt (1994), though the earlier works of O'Brien (1987) and Rootzén (1988) are also relevant. Statistical properties are explored in Smith et al. (1997) and extended to the non-stationary case in Coles et al. (1994). A parallel study in the case of Markov chain transitions that are asymptotically independent is given by Bortot & Tawn (1998).

Max-stable processes were first formalized by de Haan (1985b); see also de Haan & Pickands (1984, 1986). Only limited progress has been made in the implementation of such models for a spatial setting. Smith (1991b) gives a simple model, some of whose properties can be evaluated analytically, and Coles (1993) gives an alternative family of models that has close connections with the Poisson process models for multivariate extremes discussed in Chapter 8. Coles & Walshaw (1994) also develop a max-stable process model to describe directional dependence in wind speed measurements. A general overview is given by Coles (1994).

Latent process models are standard in other areas of spatial statistics. Replacing the GEV distribution in (9.14) with a Normal distribution having mean $\mu(r)$, and assuming the $\mu(r)$ process to be a smooth Gaussian process, leads to the standard kriging models; see Cressie (1993) for example. Diggle et al. (1998) developed computational algorithms for solving the inference problems in the non-Gaussian case, which were implemented in the extreme value setting by Coles & Casson (1999).

Appendix A
Computational Aspects

Introduction

All of the computations and graphics in this book were performed in the statistical language S-PLUS. The datasets, and many of the S-PLUS functions, are available for downloading via the internet from the URL address

http://www.maths.bris.ac.uk/~masgc/ismev/summary.html

This page will be updated on a regular basis. It currently includes:

1. Datasets in S-PLUS format;

2. S-PLUS functions to carry out the univariate analyses described in Chapters 3, 4, 6 and 7;

3. A document detailing how to use the S-PLUS functions and datasets;

4. Links to other sites that make extreme value software available, including some of the S-PLUS functions[1] used in Chapter 8.

The Univariate Functions

A brief description of the functions prepared for modeling univariate data – of either block maximum, or threshold exceedance type – is as follows:

---

[1] These functions were written by Jan Heffernan of Lancaster University.

gev.fit Function for finding maximum likelihood estimators of the GEV model. Covariate models for each of the GEV parameters are allowed, together with link functions on any of the parameters as explained in Chapter 6.

gev.diag Takes as input the output of the function gev.fit and produces diagnostic plots to check the quality of model fit.

gev.profxi Plots the profile likelihood for ξ in the GEV model.

gev.prof Plots the profile likelihood for specified return level in the GEV model.

gum.fit Function for finding maximum likelihood estimators of the Gumbel distribution, corresponding to the special case of the GEV distribution with $\xi = 0$. Covariate models and link functions for either the location or scale parameter are enabled.

gum.diag Takes as input the output of the function gum.fit and produces diagnostic plots to check the quality of model fit.

rlarg.fit Function for finding maximum likelihood estimators of the r largest order statistic model. User can specify required number of order statistics to model. Covariate models and link functions are enabled.

rlarg.diag Takes as input the output from rlarg.fit and produces probability and quantile plots for each of the r largest order statistics.

mrl.plot Function for plotting mean residual life plots.

gpd.fit Function for finding maximum likelihood estimators of the generalized Pareto distribution at specified threshold. Covariate models and link functions are enabled.

gpd.diag Takes as input the output of the function gpd.fit and produces diagnostic plots to check quality of model fit.

gpd.profxi Plots the profile likelihood for ξ in the generalized Pareto model.

gpd.prof Plots the profile likelihood for specified return level in the generalized Pareto model.

gpd.fitrange Calculates and plots maximum likelihood estimates and confidence intervals for the generalized Pareto model over a range of thresholds.

Appendix A. Computational Aspects   187

pp.fit Finds maximum likelihood estimates and standard errors for the point process model as described in Chapter 7. Covariate models and link functions are enabled for each of the model parameters, together with variable thresholds.

pp.diag Takes as input the output of the function pp.fit and produces diagnostic plots to check quality of model fit.

pp.fitrange Calculates and plots maximum likelihood estimates and confidence intervals for the point process model over a range of thresholds.

To illustrate the use of these functions, we describe an analysis of the exchange rate series between the Euro and UK sterling, similar to each of exchange rate series described in Example 1.11. This series is the contained in the dataset euroex.data. Typing[2]

```
> length(euorex.data)
[1] 975
```

confirms the length of the series as 975. A plot of the series is produced by

```
> plot(euroex.data,type='l',xlab='Day Number',
              ylab='Exchange Rate')
```

The output is shown in Fig. A.1. The transformation to log-daily returns is made as

```
euroex.ldr <- log(euroex.data[2:975])-log(euroex.data[1:974])
```

and plotted by

```
> plot(euroex.ldr,type='l',xlab='Day Number',
              ylab='Log-Daily Return')
```

This plot is shown in Fig. A.2, and suggests that the transformed series is close to stationarity.

So far this is standard S-PLUS. Further analysis requires the additional routines described above. An extreme value analysis can be based on either the threshold excess methodology of Chapter 4 or the point process model of Chapter 7. We illustrate with the former. It is convenient first to re-scale the data

```
> euroex.ldr <- 100*euroex.ldr
```

A mean residual life plot is produced by

```
> mrl.plot(euroex.ldr)
```

---

[2] We follow the convention of using the symbol > to denote the S-PLUS prompt.

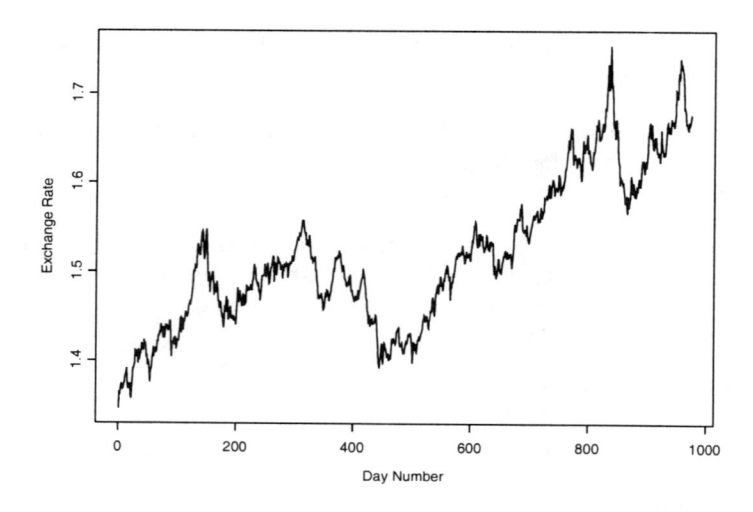

FIGURE A.1. Euro/Sterling exchange rate series.

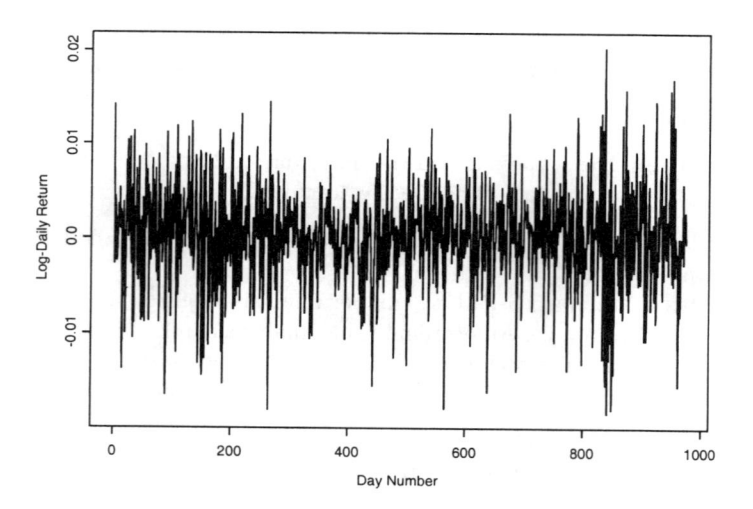

FIGURE A.2. Log-daily returns of Euro/Sterling exchange rate series.

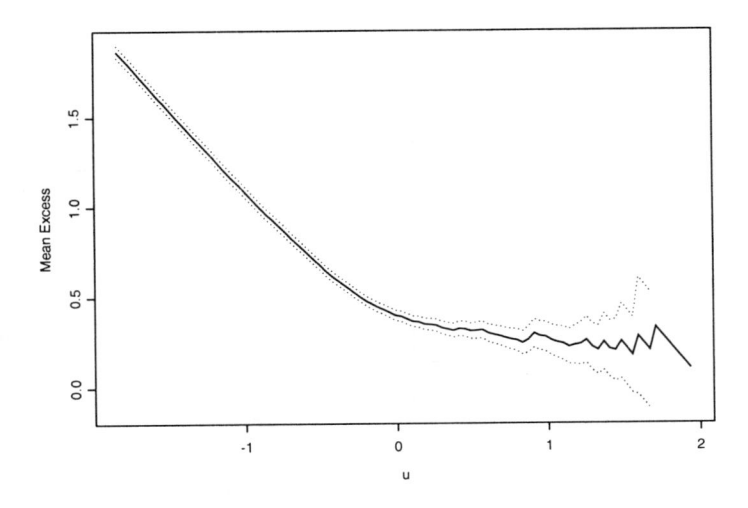

FIGURE A.3. Mean residual life plot of Euro/Sterling exchange rate log-daily returns.

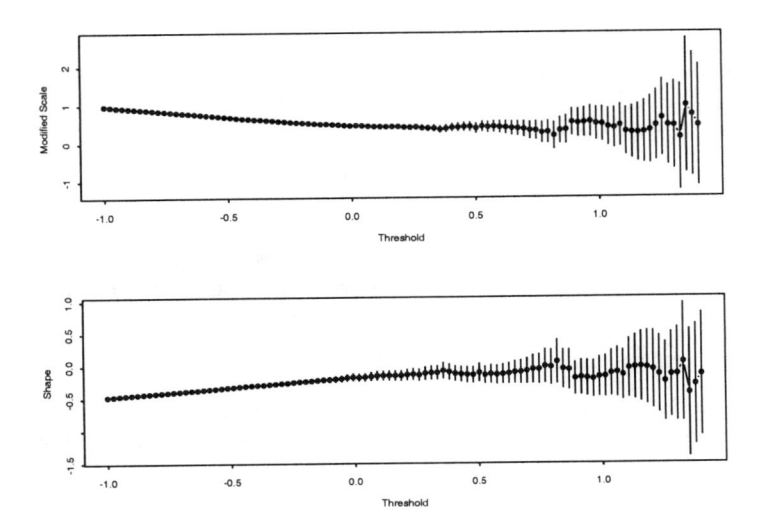

FIGURE A.4. Maximum likelihood estimates of the reparameterized generalized Pareto model as a function of threshold for Euro/Sterling exchange rate log-daily returns, and 95% confidence intervals.

190   Appendix A. Computational Aspects

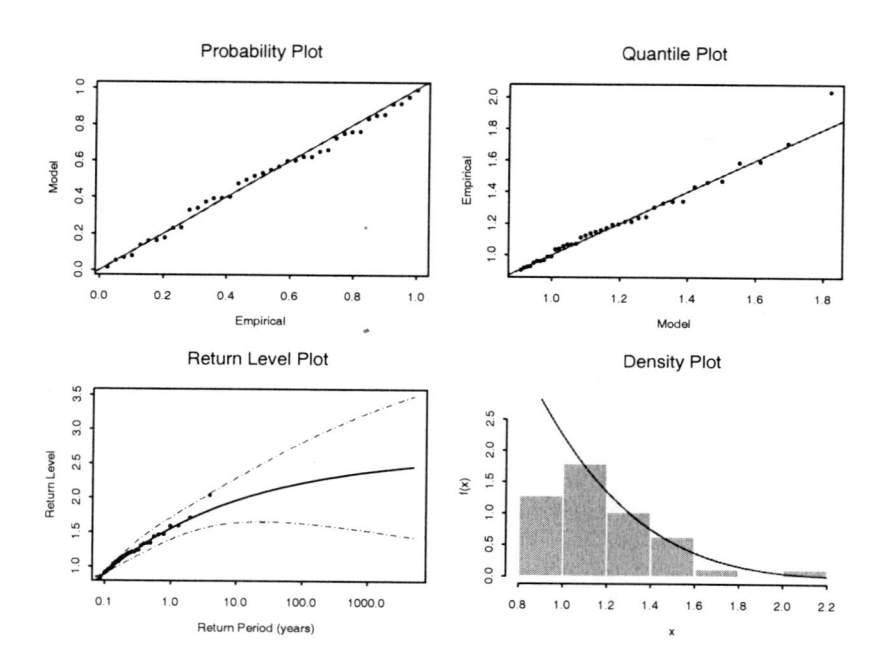

FIGURE A.5. Diagnostic plots for threshold excess analysis of Euro/Sterling exchange rate log-daily returns.

The output is shown in Fig. A.3. Approximate linearity in the plot seems to occur at a value of around $u = 0.9$. We can check how many threshold exceedances this generates by

```
> length(euroex.ldr[euroex.ldr>0.9])
[1] 39
```

The validity of the threshold $u = 0.9$ can be assessed in greater detail by checking stability with respect to u of the maximum likelihood estimates for the reparameterized model as discussed in Chapter 4:

```
> gpd.fitrange(euroex.ldr,-1,1.4,nint=100)
```

This requests estimates over the range $u = -1$ to $u = 1.4$, equally spaced so as to give 100 estimates in total. The output is shown in Fig. A.4, supporting the use of the threshold $u = 0.9$.

To fit the model at the specified threshold:

```
> euroex.gpd <- gpd.fit(euroex.ldr,0.9,npy=250)
$threshold:
[1] 0.9

$nexc:
```

```
[1] 39

$conv:
[1] T

$nllh:
[1] -9.420511

$mle:
[1]   0.3534534 -0.2015480

$rate:
[1] 0.04004107

$se:
[1] 0.07277597 0.13339979
```

The argument npy=250 is specified as there are approximately 250 trading days per year. This is important for subsequent return level calculation, which is expressed on an annual scale. In the output: threshold is the chosen threshold; nexc is the number of exceedances of that threshold; conv is a true/false indicator of whether the likelihood has been satisfactorily maximized or not; nllh is the negative log-likelihood at the maximum likelihood estimate; mle are the maximum likelihood estimates of σ and ξ respectively; rate is the proportion of points exceeding the threshold; se are the approximate standard errors of σ and ξ respectively. Diagnostics of the fitted object (which was assigned to euroex.gpd) is produced by

```
> gpd.diag(euroex.gpd)
```

The output, shown in Fig. A.5, gives little reason to doubt the validity of the generalized Pareto model, and also shows how the model extrapolates. Slight concern might be expressed that the model appears to underestimate at the top end, so that in the return level plot the largest observed value is on the bound of the corresponding confidence interval. To a large extent, this is due to the substantial uncertainty in the model which is not properly reflected in confidence intervals obtained via the delta method approximation. Better accuracy is achieved with the profile likelihood. For the shape parameter ξ,

```
> gpd.profxi(euroex.gpd,-0.5,0.3)
```

generates the plot in Fig. A.6, while for return levels corresponding to a 10-year return period,

```
> gpd.prof(euroex.gpd,m=10,npy=250,1.75,3.5)
```

gives the plot in Fig. A.7. Some trial-and-error is needed in both functions to find a suitable plotting range. Additionally, for the return level profile likelihood, it is necessary to specify the number of observations per year as npy and the desired return period as m. Fig. A.6, in particular, shows considerable asymmetry in the profile log-likelihood surface, leading to confidence intervals that are asymmetric about the maximum likelihood estimate. From the graph, the estimate is obtained as 1.97, with a 95% confidence interval – obtained at the intercept with the drawn horizontal line – of [1.76, 2.86]. It is clear that, once such asymmetries are accounted for, the model and empirical information are mutually consistent.

Finally, we can assess the evidence for non-stationarity in the series. The simplest alternative to stationarity in this model is a trend in the scale parameter σ. As discussed in Chapter 6, it is natural to build models for σ on a logarithmic scale, so as to ensure positivity. Hence, the simplest alternative model is $\log \sigma(t) = \beta_1 + \beta_2 t$, where t is an index of day number. Estimation in S-PLUS requires the construction of a matrix that includes all possible covariates. In this case, the only covariate is time, so we can set

```
> time=matrix(1:974,ncol=1)
```

which assigns the vector $(1,\ldots,974)^T$ to the object time. To fit the model:

```
> euroex.gpd2 <- gpd.fit(euroex.ldr,u=0.9,npy=250,
                         ydat=time,sigl=1,siglink=exp)
```

...

```
$nllh:
[1] -12.46977

$mle:
[1] -1.34699468   0.00082711 -0.38424075

$rate:
[1] 0.04004107

$se:
[1] 0.2253065224 0.0002391714 0.1462967335
```

The new syntax is as follows: ydat is a matrix whose columns contain the covariates; sigl is a vector listing the columns of ydat that are to be included in a linear model for σ; siglink is the inverse link to be used for modeling σ. In this way, more elaborate models can be built for σ by extending the columns of ydat, and also for ξ, by specifying shl and (if

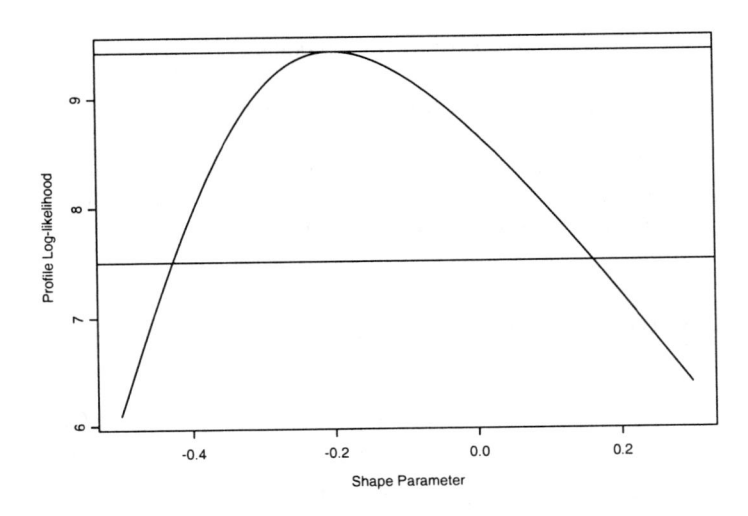

FIGURE A.6. Profile likelihood of generalized Pareto parameter ξ in threshold exceedance analysis of Euro/Sterling exchange rate log-daily returns.

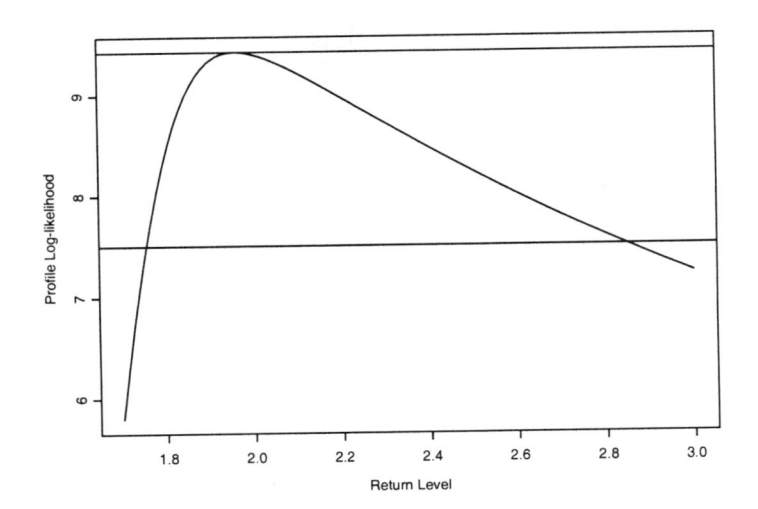

FIGURE A.7. Profile likelihood of 10-year return level in threshold exceedance analysis of Euro/Sterling exchange rate log-daily returns.

required) `shlink` in a similar format to `sigl` and `siglink`.[3] The output lists all of the sub-parameters for each parameter in turn. So, in this case, the estimated model for σ is

$$\hat{\sigma}(t) = \exp(-1.35 + 0.00083t),$$

while $\hat{\xi} = -0.384$. A comparison of the log-likelihoods from the two models, or comparison of the estimated trend parameter with its standard error, suggests that this model is an improvement on the original model, implying non-stationarity in the series. Diagnostic checks can also be made by applying `gpd.diag` to the fitted object `euroex.gpd2`.

Other Sources of Software

Other sources of software for modeling extremes are also available. Some S-PLUS functions for bivariate analyses of extremes as used in Chapter 8 of this book, together with supporting documentation, can be found at

http://www.maths.lancs.ac.uk/~currie

This software was written by Jan Heffernan of Lancaster University. The Xtremes package, made available in Reiss & Thomas (2001), enables estimation of extreme value models by a variety of alternative techniques to maximum likelihood. Closer in spirit to the main theme of this book, a further suite of S-PLUS routines, with particular routines for financial applications, is provided by Alexander McNeill at

http://www.math.ethz.ch/~mcneil/software.html

Finally, under current development by Thomas Yee of Auckland University, is a suite of S-PLUS and R functions to implement a class of models described as vector generalized additive models (VGAMs); see Yee & Wild (1996). The extreme value models form a special class of this family, and the developer is currently adapting routines to enable explicit specification of this sub-class. Once complete, the routines are likely to supersede most of the previous univariate S-PLUS routines, as they will enable both parametric and nonparametric specification of model structure for the extreme value model parameters. On completion, the routines will be available for download from

http://www.stat.auckland.ac.nz/yee/

---

[3]The syntax for the other fitting routines is similar, but with models for a location parameter μ expressed through `mul` and `mulink`.

References

AZZALINI, A. (1996). *Statistical Inference Based on the Likelihood.* Chapman and Hall, London.

BARNETT, V. (1976). The ordering of multivariate data (with discussion). *Journal of the Royal Statistical Society,* **A 139**, 318–355.

BEIRLANT, J., VYNCKIER, P., & TEUGELS, J. L. (1996). Tail index estimation, Pareto quantile plots, and regression diagnostics. *Journal of the American Statistical Association* **91**, 1659–1667.

BORTOT, P. & TAWN, J. A. (1998). Models for the extremes of Markov chains. *Biometrika* **85**, 851–867.

BROUSSARD, J. P. & BOOTH, G. G. (1998). The behaviour of extreme values in Germany's stock index futures: an application to intra-daily margin setting. *European Journal of Operational Research* **104**, 393–402.

BRUUN, J. T. & TAWN, J. A. (1998). Comparison of approaches for estimating the probability of coastal flooding. *Applied Statistics* **47**, 405–423.

BUISHAND, T. A. (1984). Bivariate extreme value data and the station-year method. *Journal of Hydrology* **69**, 77–95.

BUISHAND, T. A. (1989). Statistics of extremes in climatology. *Statistica Neerlandica* **43**, 1–30.

BUISHAND, T. A. (1991). Extreme rainfall estimation by combining data from several sites. *Hydrological Science Journal* **36**, 345–365.

CAPÉRAÀ, P., FOUGERES, A. L., & GENEST, C. (1997). A nonparametric estimation procedure for bivariate extreme value copulas. *Biometrika* **84**, 567–577.

CARTER, D. J. T. & CHALLENOR, P. G. (1981). Estimating return values of environmental parameters. *Quarterly Journal of the Royal Meteorological Society* **107**, 259–266.

CASELLA, G. & BERGER, J. O. (2001). *Statistical Inference.* Duxbury, 2nd edition.

CASTILLO, E. (1988). *Extreme Value Theory in Engineering.* Academic Press, San Diego.

CHAVEZ-DEMOULIN, V. (1999). *Two problems in environmental statistics: capture-recapture models and smooth extremal models.* PhD thesis, EPFL, Lausanne, Switzerland.

COHEN, J. P. (1988). Fitting extreme value distributions to maxima. *Sankyha, Series A* **50**, 74–97.

COLES, S. G. (1993). Regional modelling of extreme storms via max-stable processes. *Journal of the Royal Statistical Society,* **B 55**, 797–816.

COLES, S. G. (1994). Some aspects of spatial extremes. In Galambos, J., Lechner, J., & Simiu, E., editors, *Extreme Value Theory and Applications,* pages 269–282. Kluwer, Dordrecht.

COLES, S. G. & CASSON, E. A. (1999). Spatial regression models for extremes. *Extremes* **1**, 449–468.

COLES, S. G., HEFFERNAN, J., & TAWN, J. A. (1999). Dependence measures for multivariate extremes. *Extremes* **2**, 339–365.

COLES, S. G. & POWELL, E. A. (1996). Bayesian methods in extreme value modelling: a review and new developments. *International Statistical Review* **64**, 119–136.

COLES, S. G. & TAWN, J. A. (1990). Statistics of coastal flood prevention. *Philosophical Transactions of the Royal Society of London,* **A 332**, 457–476.

COLES, S. G. & TAWN, J. A. (1991). Modelling extreme multivariate events. *Journal of the Royal Statistical Society,* **B 53**, 377–392.

COLES, S. G. & TAWN, J. A. (1994). Statistical methods for multivariate extremes: an application to structural design (with discussion). *Applied Statistics* **43**, 1–48.

COLES, S. G. & TAWN, J. A. (1996a). A Bayesian analysis of extreme rainfall data. *Applied Statistics* **45**, 463–478.

COLES, S. G. & TAWN, J. A. (1996b). Modelling extremes of the areal rainfall process. *Journal of the Royal Statistical Society,* **B 58**, 329–347.

COLES, S. G., TAWN, J. A., & SMITH, R. L. (1994). A seasonal Markov model for extremely low temperatures. *Environmetrics* **5**, 221–239.

COLES, S. G. & WALSHAW, D. (1994). Directional modelling of extreme wind speeds. *Applied Statistics* **43**, 139–157.

COX, D. R. & HINKLEY, D. V. (1974). *Theoretical Statistics.* Chapman and Hall, London.

COX, D. R. & ISHAM, V. (1980). *Point Processes.* Chapman and Hall, London.

CRESSIE, N. A. C. (1993). *Statistics for Spatial Data.* Wiley, Chichester.

CROWDER, M. J., KIMBER, A. C., & SMITH, R. L. (1991). *Statistical Analysis of Reliability Data*. Kluwer, Amsterdam.

DAHAN, E. & MENDELSON, H. (2001). An extreme value model of concept testing. *Management Science* **47**, 102–116.

DALES, M. Y. & REED, D. W. (1988). Regional flood and storm hazard assessment. Technical Report 102, Institute of Hydrology, Wallingford, UK.

DAVISON, A. C. (1984). Modelling excesses over high thresholds, with an application. In Tiago de Oliveira, J., editor, *Statistical Extremes and Applications*, pages 461–482. Reidel, Dordrecht.

DAVISON, A. C. & RAMESH, N. I. (2000). Smoothing sample extremes. *Journal of the Royal Statistical Society*, **B 62**, 191–208.

DAVISON, A. C. & SMITH, R. L. (1990). Models for exceedances over high thresholds (with discussion). *Journal of the Royal Statistical Society*, **B 52**, 393–442.

DAWSON, T. H. (2000). Maximum wave crests in heavy seas. *Journal of Offshore Mechanics and Arctic Engineering – Transactions of the AMSE* **122**, 222–224.

DE HAAN, L. (1985a). Extremes in higher dimensions: the model and some statistics. *Bulletin of the Institute of International Statistics* **51**, 185–192. Proceedings of the 45th Session of the I.S.I.

DE HAAN, L. (1985b). A spectral representation for max–stable processes. *Annals of Probability* **12**, 1194–1204.

DE HAAN, L. (1990). Fighting the arch-enemy with mathematics. *Statistica Neerlandica* **44**, 45–68.

DE HAAN, L. & PICKANDS, J. (1984). A spectral representation for stationary min-stable stochastic processes. *Stochastic Processes and their Applications* **17**, 26–27.

DE HAAN, L. & PICKANDS, J. (1986). Stationary min-stable stochastic processes. *Probability Theory and Related Fields* **72**, 477–492.

DE HAAN, L. & RESNICK, S. I. (1977). Limit theory for multivariate sample extremes. *Zeit. Wahrscheinl.-theorie* **40**, 317–337.

DE HAAN, L., RESNICK, S. I., ROOTZÉN, H., & DE VRIES, C. G. (1989). Extremal behaviour of solutions to a stochastic difference equation with applications to ARCH processes. *Stochastic Processes and their Applications* **32**, 213–224.

DEHEUVELS, P. & TIAGO DE OLIVEIRA, J. (1989). On the nonparametric estimation of the bivariate extreme value distributions. *Statistics and Probability Letters* **8**, 315–323.

DEKKERS, A. L. M. & DE HAAN, L. (1993). Optimal choice of sample fraction in extreme value estimation. *Journal of Multivariate Analysis* **47**, 173–195.

DIEBOLD, F. X., SCHUERMANN, T., & STROUGHAIR, J. D. (1997). Pitfalls and opportunities in the use of extreme value theory in risk management. *Advances in Computational Management Science* **2**, 3–12.

DIGGLE, P. J., TAWN, J. A., & MOYEED, R. A. (1998). Non-linear geostatistics (with discussion). *Applied Statistics* **47**, 299–350.

DIXON, M. J. & TAWN, J. A. (1999). The effect of non-stationarity on extreme sea-level estimation. *Applied Statistics* **48**, 135–151.

DREES, H., DE HAAN, L., & RESNICK, S. (2000). How to make a Hill plot. *Annals of Statistics* **28**, 254–274.

DUNNE, J. F. & GHANBARI, M. (2001). Efficient extreme value prediction for nonlinear beam vibrations using measured random response histories. *Nonlinear Dynamics* **24**, 71–101.

EINMAHL, J. H. J., DE HAAN, L., & SINHA, A. K. (1997). Estimating the spectral measure of an extreme value distribution. *Stochastic Processes and their Applications* **70**, 143–171.

EINMAHL, J. H. J., DE HAAN, L., & XIN, H. (1993). Estimating a multidimensional extreme value distribution. *Journal of Multivariate Analysis* **47**, 35–47.

EMBRECHTS, P., KLÜPPELBURG, C., & MIKOSCH, T. (1998). *Modelling Extremal Events for Insurance and Finance*. Springer, New York.

FISHER, R. A. & TIPPETT, L. H. C. (1928). On the estimation of the frequency distributions of the largest or smallest member of a sample. *Proceedings of the Cambridge Philosophical Society* **24**, 180–190.

FITZGERALD, D. L. (1989). Single station and regional analysis of daily rainfall extremes. *Stochastic Hydrology and Hydraulics* **3**, 281–292.

GALAMBOS, J. (1987). *The Asymptotic Theory of Extreme Order Statistics*. Krieger, Florida, 2nd edition. 1st edition published by Wiley, 1978.

GALAMBOS, J. (1995). The development of the mathematical theory of extremes in the past half-century. *Theory of Probability and its Applications* **39**, 234–248.

GALAMBOS, J., LEIGH, S., & SIMIU, E. (1994). *Extreme Value Theory and Applications*. Kluwer, Amsterdam.

GILKS, W. R., RICHARDSON, S., & SPIEGELHALTER, D. J. (1996). *Markov Chain Monte Carlo in Practice*. Chapman and Hall, London.

GNEDENKO, B. V. (1943). Sur la distribution limite du terme maximum d'une série aléatoire. *Annals of Mathematics* **44**, 423–453.

GRADY, A. M. (1992). Modeling daily minimum temperatures: an application of the threshold method. In Zwiers, F., editor, *Proceedings of the 5th International Meeting on Statistical Climatology*, pages 319–324, Toronto. Canadian Climate Centre.

GRIMMETT, G. R. & STIRZAKER, D. R. (1992). *Probability and Random Processes*. Oxford University Press, Oxford, 2nd edition.

GUMBEL, E. J. (1958). *Statistics of Extremes*. Columbia University Press, New York.

GUMBEL, E. J. (1960). Distributions de valeurs extremes en plusieurs dimensions. *Publications of the Institute of Statistics of the University of Paris* **9**, 171–173.

HALL, P. & TAJVIDI, N. (2000a). Distribution and dependence function

estimation for bivariate extreme value distributions. *Bernoulli* **6**, 835–844.
HALL, P. & TAJVIDI, N. (2000b). Nonparametric analysis of temporal trend when fitting parametric models to extreme value data. *Statistical Science* **15**, 153–167.
HARRIS, R. I. (2001). The accuracy of design values predicted from extreme value analysis. *Journal of Wind Engineering and Industrial Aerodynamics* **89**, 153–164.
HENERY, R. J. (1984). An extreme value model for predicting the results of horse races. *Applied Statistics* **33**, 125–133.
HILL, B. M. (1975). A simple general approach to inference about the tail of a distribution. *Annals of Statistics* **3**, 1163–1174.
HO, L. C., BURRIDGE, P., CADLE, J., & THEOBALD, M. (2000). Value-at-risk: applying the extreme value approach to Asian markets in the recent financial turmoil. *Pacific Basin Finance Journal* **8**, 249–275.
HOSKING, J. R. M. (1984). Testing whether the shape parameter is zero in the generalized extreme value distribution. *Biometrika* **71**, 367–374.
HOSKING, J. R. M. (1985). Maximum likelihood estimation of the parameters of the generalized extreme value distribution. *Applied Statistics* **34**, 301–310.
HOSKING, J. R. M., WALLIS, J. R., & WOOD, E. F. (1985). Estimation of the generalized extreme value distribution by the method of probability-weighted moments. *Technometrics* **27**, 251–261.
HSING, T. (1989). Extreme value theory for multivariate stationary sequences. *Journal of Multivariate Analysis* **29**, 274–291.
HÜSLER, J. (1984). Frost data: a case study on extreme values of non-stationary sequences. In Tiago de Oliveria, J., editor, *Statistical Extremes and Applications*, pages 513–520. Reidel, Dordrecht.
HÜSLER, J. (1986). Extreme values of non-stationary random sequences. *Journal of Applied Probability* **23**, 937–950.
HÜSLER, J. (1996). Multivariate option price models and extremes. *Communications in Statistics: Theory and Methods* **25**, 853–870.
JENKINSON, A. F. (1955). The frequency distribution of the annual maximum (or minimum) values of meteorological events. *Quarterly Journal of the Royal Meteorological Society* **81**, 158–172.
JOE, H. (1989). Families of min-stable multivariate exponential and multivariate extreme value distributions. *Statistics and Probability Letters* **9**, 75–81.
JOE, H. (1994). Multivariate extreme value distributions with applications to environmental data. *Canadian Journal of Statistics* **22**, 47–64.
JOE, H., SMITH, R. L., & WEISSMAN, I. (1992). Bivariate threshold methods for extremes. *Journal of the Royal Statistical Society,* **B 54**, 171–183.
KAWAS, M. L. & MOREIRA, R. G. (2001). Characterization of product quality attributes of tortilla chips during the frying process. *Journal of*

Food Engineering **47**, 97–107.

KOEDIJK, K. D. & KOOL, C. J. M. (1992). Tail estimates of east European exchange rates. *Journal of Business Economics and Statistics* **10**, 83–96.

KOTZ, S. & NADARAJAH, S. (2000). *Extreme Value Distributions: Theory and Applications*. Imperial College Press, London.

LAVENDA, B. H. & CIPOLLONE, E. (2000). Extreme value statistics and thermodynamics of earthquakes: aftershock sequences. *Annali di geofisica* **43**, 967–982.

LAYCOCK, P. J., COTTIS, R. A., & SCARF, P. A. (1990). Extrapolation of extreme pit depths on space and time. *Journal of the Electrochemical Society* **137**, 64–99.

LEADBETTER, M. R. (1983). Extremes and local dependence in stationary-sequences. *Zeit. Wahrscheinl.-theorie* **65**, 291–306.

LEADBETTER, M. R., LINDGREN, G., & ROOTZÉN, H. (1983). *Extremes and Related Properties of Random Sequences and Series*. Springer Verlag, New York.

LEADBETTER, M. R. & ROOTZÉN, H. (1988). Extremal theory for stochastic processes. *Annals of Probability* **16**, 431–478.

LEADBETTER, M. R., WEISSMAN, I., DE HAAN, L., & ROOTZÉN, H. (1989). On clustering of high levels in statistically stationary series. In Sansom, J., editor, *Proceedings of the 4th International Meeting on Statistical Climatology*. New Zealand Meteorological Service, Wellington.

LEDFORD, A. & TAWN, J. A. (1996). Statistics for near independence in multivariate extreme values. *Biometrika* **83**, 169–187.

LEDFORD, A. & TAWN, J. A. (1997). Modelling dependence within joint tail regions. *Journal of the Royal Statistical Society,* **B 59**, 475–499.

LEDFORD, A. & TAWN, J. A. (1998). Concomitant tail behaviour for extremes. *Advances in Applied Probability* **30**, 197–215.

LONGIN, F. M. (2000). From value at risk to stress testing: the extreme value approach. *Journal of Banking and Finance* **24**, 1097–1130.

MCNEIL, A. J. & FREY, R. (2000). Estimation of tail-related risk measures for heteroscedastic financial time series: an extreme value approach. *Journal of Empirical Finance* **7**, 271–300.

MCNULTY, P. J., SCHEICK, L. Z., ROTH, D. R., DAVIS, M. G., & TORTORA, M. R. S. (2000). First failure predictions for EPROMs of the type flown on the MPTB satellite. *IEEE Transactions on Nuclear Science* **47**, 2237–2243.

MOLE, N., ANDERSON, C. W., NADARAJAH, S., & WRIGHT, C. (1995). A generalized Pareto distribution model for high concentrations in short-range atmospheric dispersion. *Environmetrics* **6**, 595–606.

MOORE, R. J. (1987). Combined regional flood frequency analysis and regression on catchment characteristics by maximum likelihood estimation. In Singh, V. P., editor, *Regional Flood Frequency Analysis*, pages 119–131. Reidel, Dordrecht.

MORTON, I. D., BOWERS, J., & MOULD, G. (1997). Estimating return period wave heights and wind speeds using a seasonal point process model. *Coastal Engineering* **31**, 305–326.

O'BRIEN, G. L. (1987). Extreme values for stationary and Markov sequences. *Annals of Probability* **15**, 281–291.

O'HAGAN, A. (1994). *Kendall's Theory of Advanced Statistics*, volume 2B. Arnold, London.

PAULI, F. & COLES, S. G. (2001). Penalized likelihood inference in extreme value analyses. *Journal of Applied Statistics* **28**, 547–560.

PERFEKT, R. (1994). Extremal behaviour of stationary Markov chains with applications. *Annals of Applied Probability* **4**, 529–548.

PICKANDS, J. (1971). The two-dimensional poisson process and extremal processes. *Journal of Applied Probability* **8**, 745–756.

PICKANDS, J. (1975). Statistical inference using extreme order statistics. *Annals of Statistics* **3**, 119–131.

PICKANDS, J. (1981). Multivariate extreme value distributions. In *Proceedings of the 43rd Session of the I.S.I.*, pages 859–878, The Hague. International Statistical Institute.

PRESCOTT, P. & WALDEN, A. T. (1980). Maximum likelihood estimation of the parameters of the generalized extreme value distribution. *Biometrika* **67**, 723–724.

PRESCOTT, P. & WALDEN, A. T. (1983). Maximum likelihood estimation of the parameters of the three-parameter generalized extreme value distribution from censored samples. *Journal of Statistical Computation and Simulation* **16**, 241–250.

REISS, R.-D. & THOMAS, M. (2001). *Statistical Analysis of Extreme Values with Applications to Insurance, Finance, Hydrology and Other Fields*. Birkhauser Verlag AG, 2nd edition.

RESNICK, S. I. (1987). *Extreme Values, Regular Variation, and Point Processes*. Springer Verlag, New York.

ROBERTS, S. J. (2000). Extreme value statistics for novelty detection in biomedical data processing. *IEE Proceedings – Science Measurement and Technology* **147**, 363–367.

ROBINSON, M. E. & TAWN, J. A. (1995). Statistics for exceptional athletics records. *Applied Statistics* **44**, 499–511.

ROBINSON, M. E. & TAWN, J. A. (1997). Statistics for extreme sea currents. *Applied Statistics* **46**, 183–205.

ROBINSON, M. E. & TAWN, J. A. (2000). Extremal analysis of processes observed at different frequencies. *Journal of the Royal Statistical Society*, **B 62**, 117–135.

ROOTZÉN, H. (1986). Extreme value theory for moving average processes. *Annals of Probability* **14**, 612–652.

ROOTZÉN, H. (1988). Maxima and exceedances of stationary Markov chains. *Advances in Applied Probability* **20**, 371–390.

ROSEN, G. & COHEN, A. (1994). Extreme percentile regression. In *Sta-*

tistical Theory and Computational Aspects of Smoothing: Proceedings of the COMPSTAT '94 satellite meeting, pages 200–214. Physica-Verlag, Heidelberg.

SCARF, P. A. & LAYCOCK, P. J. (1996). Estimation of extremes in corrosion engineering. *Journal of Applied Statistics* **23**, 621–643.

SIBUYA, M. (1960). Bivariate extreme statistics. *Ann. Inst. Statist. Math.* **11**, 195–210.

SILVEY, S. D. (1970). *Statistical Inference*. Chapman and Hall, London.

SMITH, R. L. (1984). Threshold methods for sample extremes. In Tiago de Oliveira, J., editor, *Statistical Extremes and Applications*, pages 621–638. Reidel, Dordrecht.

SMITH, R. L. (1985). Maximum likelihood estimation in a class of non-regular cases. *Biometrika* **72**, 67–90.

SMITH, R. L. (1986). Extreme value theory based on the r largest annual events. *Journal of Hydrology* **86**, 27–43.

SMITH, R. L. (1989a). Extreme value analysis of environmental time series: an example based on ozone data (with discussion). *Statistical Science* **4**, 367–393.

SMITH, R. L. (1989b). A survey of nonregular problems. In *Proceedings of the 47th meeting of the I.S.I.*, pages 353–372. International Statistical Institute.

SMITH, R. L. (1991a). Extreme value theory. In Ledermann, W., editor, *Handbook of Applicable Mathematics*, volume 7, chapter 14, pages 437–472. Wiley, Chichester.

SMITH, R. L. (1991b). Spatial extremes and max-stable processes. Technical report, University of North Carolina.

SMITH, R. L. (1992). The extremal index for a Markov chain. *Journal of Applied Probability* **29**, 37–45.

SMITH, R. L. (1994). Multivariate threshold methods. In Galambos, J., Lechner, J., & Simiu, E., editors, *Extreme Value Theory and Applications*, pages 225–248. Kluwer, Dordrecht.

SMITH, R. L. (1995). Likelihood and modified likelihood estimation for distributions with unknown endpoints. In Balakrishnan, N., editor, *Recent Advances in Life-Testing and Reliabilty. A Volume in Honor of Alonzo Clifford Cohen, Jr.*, chapter 24, pages 455–474. CRC Press, Boca Raton.

SMITH, R. L. (1999). Bayesian and frequentist approaches to parametric predictive inference (with discussion). In Bernardo, J. M., Berger, J. O., Dawid, A. P., & Smith, A. F. M., editors, *Bayesian Statistics 6*, pages 589–612. Oxford University Press.

SMITH, R. L. & NAYLOR, J. C. (1987). A comparison of maximum likelihood and Bayesian estimators for the three-parameter Weibull distribution. *Applied Statistics* **36**, 358–369.

SMITH, R. L., TAWN, J. A., & COLES, S. G. (1997). Markov chain models for threshold exceedances. *Biometrika* **84**, 249–268.

SMITH, R. L., TAWN, J. A., & YUEN, H. K. (1990). Statistics of multi-

variate extremes. *International Statistical Review* **58**, 47–58.
SMITH, R. L. & WEISSMAN, I. (1994). Estimating the extremal index. *Journal of the Royal Statistical Society, B* **56**, 515–528.
TAWN, J. A. (1988a). Bivariate extreme value theory: models and estimation. *Biometrika* **75**, 397–415.
TAWN, J. A. (1988b). An extreme value theory model for dependent observations. *Journal of Hydrology* **101**, 227–250.
TAWN, J. A. (1990). Modelling multivariate extreme value distributions. *Biometrika* **77**, 245–253.
TAWN, J. A. (1992). Estimating probabilities of extreme sea-levels. *Applied Statistics* **41**, 77–93.
TAWN, J. A. (1994). Applications of multivariate extremes. In Galambos, J., Lechner, J., & Simiu, E., editors, *Extreme Value Theory and Applications*, pages 249–268. Kluwer, Dordrecht.
TAWN, J. A. & VASSIE, J. M. (1989). Extreme sea levels – the joint probabilities method revisited and revised. *Proceedings of the Institute of Civil Engineers Part 2 – Research and Theory* **87**, 429–442.
TAWN, J. A. & VASSIE, J. M. (1990). Spatial transfer of extreme sea-level data for use in the revised joint probability method. *Proceedings of the Institute of Civil Engineers Part 2 – Research and Theory* **89**, 433–438.
THOMPSON, M. L., REYNOLDS, J., COX, L. H., GUTTORP, P., & SAMPSON, P. D. (2001). A review of statistical methods for the meteorological adjustment of tropospheric ozone. *Atmospheric Environment* **35**, 617–630.
TIAGO DE OLIVEIRA, J. (1984a). Bivariate models for extremes. In *Statistical Extremes and Applications*, pages 131–153. Reidel, Dordrecht.
TIAGO DE OLIVEIRA, J. (1984b). *Statistical Extremes and Applications*. Reidel, Dordrecht.
TRYON, R. G. & CRUSE, T. A. (2000). Probabilistic mesomechanics for high cycle fatigue life prediction. *Journal of Engineering Materials and Technolgy – Transactions of the AMSE* **122**, 209–214.
VENABLES, W. N. & RIPLEY, B. D. (1997). *Statistical Modelling with S-PLUS*. Springer, New York, 2nd edition.
VON MISES, R. (1954). La distribution de la plus grande de n valeurs. In *Selected Papers, Volume II*, pages 271–294. American Mathematical Society, Providence, RI.
WALSHAW, D. (1994). Getting the most from your extreme wind data: a step by step guide. *Journal of Research of the National Institute of Standards and Technology* **99**, 399–411.
WALSHAW, D. (2000). Modelling extreme wind speeds in regions prone to hurricanes. *Applied Statistics* **49**, 51–62.
WALSHAW, D. & ANDERSON, C. W. (2000). A model for extreme wind gusts. *Applied Statistics* **49**, 499–508.
WEISSMAN, I. (1978). Estimation of parameters and quantiles based on the k largest observations. *Journal of the American Statistical Association*

73, 812–815.

WIGGINS, J. B. (1992). Estimating the volatility of S-and-P 500 futures using the extreme value method. *Journal of Futures Markets* **12**, 265–273.

YEE, T. W. & WILD, C. J. (1996). Vector generalized additive models. *Journal of the Royal Statistical Society,* **B 58**, 481–493.

ZWIERS, F. W. (1987). An extreme value analysis of wind speeds at 5 Canadian locations. *Journal of the Canadian Statistical Society* **15**, 317–327.

ZWIERS, F. W. & ROSS, W. H. (1991). An alternative approach to the extreme value analysis of rainfall data. *Atmospheric Ocean* **29**, 437–461.

Index

$\bar{\chi}$ 164–166
χ 163, 164, 166

Asymptotic independence 163–166, 168, 182

Bayes' theorem 170
Bayesian inference 169–177, 182
– of extremes 172–177
Bias 28
Bilogistic model *see* Bivariate extreme value distribution, bilogistic model
Bivariate extreme value distribution 144–148, 156, 157, 163, 164
– bilogistic model 147, 161
– diagnostics 165
– diagnostics for 165–166
– Dirichlet model 147, 161
– likelihood function 148–150
– logistic model 146, 148, 161, 166
Bivariate threshold excess model
– asymptotic distribution 154–156
– likelihood inference 155

Central limit theorem 26, 29, 47

Componentwise maxima 143, 147, 157
Computation 185
Conditional density function 23
Confidence interval 29
Convergence in distribution 26
Correlation 24
Covariance 24
Covariate 107, 108, 113

$D(u_n)$ condition 93, 98
Datasets
– annual maximum wind speeds 11
– daily rainfall 9, 84–86, 119, 134
– Dow Jones Index 11, 86–90, 103
– engine failure times 38–43
– Euro/sterling exchange rates 187–194
– exchange rate series 13, 161–163, 166
– Fremantle sea-levels 5, 105, 109, 111–114, 148–151
– glass fiber strength 5, 64–66
– oceanographic variables 13, 158–161, 166

206   Index

- Port Pirie sea-levels   4, 59–64, 106, 111, 148–151, 173–177
- race times   7, 114–116
- Venice sea-levels   8, 67, 69–72, 117–118
- Wooster minimum temperature series   10, 99–101, 106, 119–122, 136–141

Declustering   99, 100, 103, 177, 178
Delta method   see Likelihood, delta method
Deviance statistic   35
Directional dependence   182
Dirichlet model   see Bivariate extreme value distribution, Dirichlet model

El Niño   7, 113
Empirical distribution function   36
Examples   see Datasets
- daily rainfall threshold excess analysis   85
Expectation   20
Extremal index   97, 98, 103
Extremal types theorem   46–49
Extremal types theorem for minima   53
Extreme values in non-stationary sequences   105–122
Extreme values in stationary sequences   92–104

Fréchet distribution   47, 94, 143, 148, 155, 158, 180

Generalized linear models   108
Generalized Pareto distribution   75, 76, 78, 83, 84, 86, 88, 90, 99, 101, 106, 111, 119, 132, 134, 177
- return level plot   84
GEV distribution   47, 48, 50, 53, 75, 76, 93, 96–98, 105, 107, 108, 110, 111, 113, 131, 144, 145, 147, 172, 182, 183
- diagnostics   57–59
- inference   54
- likelihood inference   55, 56, 108
- probability plot   see Probability plot, for GEV distribution
- profile likelihood   57

- quantile plot   see Quantile plot, for GEV distribution, 58
- quantiles   49, 56
- return level plot   see Return level plot
- return levels   56–58, 65
GEV distribution for minima   53
Gumbel distribution   47, 48
- likelihood inference   55, 109

Independence   23
Inverse-link function   107

Joint density function   22
Joint distribution function   22

Latent process models   181, 182
Likelihood
- delta method   32, 33, 56, 82, 83
- deviance function   33
- - asymptotic properties   34
- expected information matrix   32
- likelihood function   30
- likelihood ratio test   35, 109
- log-likelihood function   30
- maximum likelihood   30
- - asymptotic normality   31, 32
- maximum likelihood estimator   31
- - asymptotic normality   31, 57
- observed information matrix   32
- profile likelihood   34
- - asymptotic properties   35
Logistic model   see Bivariate extreme value distribution, logistic model

Marginal density function   23
Markov chain   25, 171, 178, 182
- extremal index   178
- extremal properties   177, 178
Markov chain Monte Carlo   171–173, 182
Max-stability   49, 50, 145
Max-stable processes   179, 180, 182
- Gaussian model   181
- spectral representation   180, 181
Maximum likelihood   see Likelihood, maximum likelihood
MCMC   see Markov chain Monte Carlo

Index

Mean residual life plot 79
Mean-square error 28
Model choice 64
Model diagnostics 36
Model selection 35
Multivariate distributions 22–24
- mutivariate normal distribution 24
Multivariate extreme value distribution *see* Bivariate extreme value distribution
Multivariate extremes 142–168

Non-stationarity *see* Extreme values in non-stationary sequences
Nonparametric techniques 167

Order statistics 66
- limit distribution 66–68, 141

Parameter estimation 28
Perfect dependence 145
Pivot 29
Point process 124–126
- bivariate extreme value model *see* Poisson process, limit for bivariate extremes
- convergence 128
- extreme value model *see* Poisson process, limit for extremes
- intensity measure 125
Poisson process 125
- likelihood function 126–128, 134, 135
- limit for bivariate extremes 156
-- likelihood inference 158
-- modeling 158, 161
- limit for extremes 128, 129, 131–133, 138, 141
-- modeling 132–134
-- return levels 137, 140
- non-homogeneous 125, 126
Prediction 170
- predictive distribution 171, 173
Probability density function 20
Probability distribution
- binomial distribution 129
- binomial distribution 21
- chi-squared distribution 22

- exponential distribution 76
- normal distribution 21
- Poisson distribution 21, 129
Probability distribution function 20
Probability plot 37
- for r largest order statistic model 72
- for Generalized Pareto distribution 84, 86, 88
- for GEV distribution 58, 62, 65
- for non-stationary generalized Pareto model 111
- for non-stationary GEV model 110
Profile likelihood *see* Likelihood, profile likelihood

Quantile plot 37
- for r largest order statistic model 72
- for generalized Pareto distribution 84, 86, 88
- for GEV distribution 58, 62, 65
- for non-stationary generalized Pareto model 111
- for non-stationary GEV model 110

r largest order statistic model 66–72, 117–118, 131, 141
- diagnostics 70
- inference 69
Random process 25
Random variables 19
Return level 49, 173
- plot 49, 58, 59, 81, 103
Return level plot 62, 66, 88
Return period 49

S-PLUS 185–194
Sample Maxima 45
Sample maxima
- asymptotic distribution 46, 48–50, 131
Sample minima 52
- asymptotic distribution 53
Seasonality 106, 107, 120
Southern Oscillation Index 7, 107, 108, 113

Spatial extremes 179
Standard deviation 20
Standard error 28
Stationary sequence 25
– extremes *see* Extreme values in stationary sequences
Structure variable 150, 151, 156
– return levels 150, 151, 153

Threshold excess model 98, 177
– asymptotic distribution 75, 131, 132, 154
– dependent observations 99
– diagnostics 84
– likelihood inference 80, 81, 135
– profile likelihood 82
– return levels 81, 82, 84, 101, 103
– threshold selection 78, 83, 122
Trends 106, 107, 109, 111, 114, 118, 119, 150

Variance 20
Variance-covariance matrix 24
Vector generalized additive models 194
VGAMs *see* Vector generalized additive models

Weibull distribution 47

Xtremes 194

Springer Series in Statistics *(continued from p. ii)*

Knottnerus: Sample Survey Theory: Some Pythagorean Perspectives.
Kolen/Brennan: Test Equating: Methods and Practices.
Kotz/Johnson (Eds.): Breakthroughs in Statistics Volume I.
Kotz/Johnson (Eds.): Breakthroughs in Statistics Volume II.
Kotz/Johnson (Eds.): Breakthroughs in Statistics Volume III.
Küchler/Sørensen: Exponential Families of Stochastic Processes.
Le Cam: Asymptotic Methods in Statistical Decision Theory.
Le Cam/Yang: Asymptotics in Statistics: Some Basic Concepts, 2nd edition.
Liu: Monte Carlo Strategies in Scientific Computing.
Longford: Models for Uncertainty in Educational Testing.
Manski: Partial Identification of Probability Distributions.
Mielke/Berry: Permutation Methods: A Distance Function Approach.
Pan/Fang: Growth Curve Models and Statistical Diagnostics.
Parzen/Tanabe/Kitagawa: Selected Papers of Hirotugu Akaike.
Politis/Romano/Wolf: Subsampling.
Ramsay/Silverman: Applied Functional Data Analysis: Methods and Case Studies.
Ramsay/Silverman: Functional Data Analysis.
Rao/Toutenburg: Linear Models: Least Squares and Alternatives.
Reinsel: Elements of Multivariate Time Series Analysis, 2nd edition.
Rosenbaum: Observational Studies, 2nd edition.
Rosenblatt: Gaussian and Non-Gaussian Linear Time Series and Random Fields.
Särndal/Swensson/Wretman: Model Assisted Survey Sampling.
Schervish: Theory of Statistics.
Shao/Tu: The Jackknife and Bootstrap.
Simonoff: Smoothing Methods in Statistics.
Singpurwalla and Wilson: Statistical Methods in Software Engineering:
    Reliability and Risk.
Small: The Statistical Theory of Shape.
Sprott: Statistical Inference in Science.
Stein: Interpolation of Spatial Data: Some Theory for Kriging.
Taniguchi/Kakizawa: Asymptotic Theory of Statistical Inference for Time Series.
Tanner: Tools for Statistical Inference: Methods for the Exploration of Posterior
    Distributions and Likelihood Functions, 3rd edition.
van der Laan: Unified Methods for Censored Longitudinal Data and Causality.
van der Vaart/Wellner: Weak Convergence and Empirical Processes: With
    Applications to Statistics.
Verbeke/Molenberghs: Linear Mixed Models for Longitudinal Data.
Weerahandi: Exact Statistical Methods for Data Analysis.
West/Harrison: Bayesian Forecasting and Dynamic Models, 2nd edition.